Praise for

'This book is a portal; open its pages, and you cross a threshold. Through incantation, mystical prompts, devotional practice, and luscious truth-telling, Lisa Lister offers us a sacred dissent, a holy revolution, a return to true power, to live fully, audaciously, from the body, from the source of love and beauty within us.'

MEGGAN WATTERSON, *WALL STREET JOURNAL* BEST-SELLING AUTHOR OF *MARY MAGDALENE REVEALED*

'I love Lisa. I love everything she writes. I love her voice, her way, her magic.'

CARRIE ANNE MOSS, ACTRESS AND FOUNDER OF ANNAPURNA LIVING

'Lisa is the ultimate nurturer, gently guiding us all back to remembrance. She is a fierce, unwavering force of nature, of feminine power, of love.'

LEANN RIMES CIBRIAN, SINGER-SONGWRITER, GRAMMY AWARD WINNER, AND FOUNDER OF SOUL OF EVERLE

'Lisa Lister is a badass leader of all things feminine.'

REBECCA CAMPBELL, BEST-SELLING AUTHOR OF *RISE SISTER RISE*

'Lisa is so full of womanly wisdom; she completely blows my mind.'

DENISE DUFFIELD-THOMAS, BEST-SELLING AUTHOR OF *LUCKY BITCH*

'Lisa's medicine saved me. In a very real way. Her work didn't give me answers. It gave me a map, hard truths delivered with love and humour, and the provisions I would need to take the journey to find the place long since forgotten. It gave me her compass until I could find my own.'

LEANNE BEST, ACTRESS

'Lisa Lister is the woman we all wish we were lucky enough to have as our sister.'

'Lisa is one of those rare human beings who not only teaches truth and vitality and vulnerability and divinity, but actually *embodies* it. I love her work. I love her.'

'Lisa Lister's work is like the key that unlocks an ancient door that leads you into a fantasy world that you'd always dreamed about, but had almost given up believing in. Her writing – like her – is bold, bright, beautiful and lovingly provokes the reader to embrace the fullness of their being; of wanting and asking for more and never apologizing for being too much. Reading her books feels like softening into Mama Earth's loving embrace, being held, and then being reminded that I am her and she is me.'

'In a world of bossy "self-help" and Instagram "spirituality," Lisa is the real deal. She brings something different, much-needed, and nothing short of life-changing. She is wise and wonderful; her work is genuinely authentic and from the heart.'

venus

**A Sacred Path. A Feminine Frequency.
A Sensual Love Affair with Life.**

venus
venus
venus
venus

LISA LISTER

HAY HOUSE

Carlsbad, California • New York City
London • Sydney • New Delhi

Published in the United Kingdom by:
Hay House UK Ltd, The Sixth Floor, Watson House,
54 Baker Street, London W1U 7BU
Tel: +44 (0)20 3927 7290; www.hayhouse.co.uk

Published in the United States of America by:
Hay House LLC, PO Box 5100, Carlsbad, CA 92018-5100
Tel: (1) 760 431 7695 or (800) 654 5126; www.hayhouse.com

Published in Australia by:
Hay House Australia Publishing Pty Ltd,
18/36 Ralph St, Alexandria NSW 2015
Tel: (61) 2 9669 4299; www.hayhouse.com.au

Published in India by:
Hay House Publishers (India) Pvt Ltd, Muskaan Complex,
Plot No.3, B-2, Vasant Kunj, New Delhi 110 070
Tel: (91) 11 4176 1620; www.hayhouse.co.in

A catalogue record for this book is available from the British Library.

Tradepaper ISBN: 978-1-4019-7399-5
E-book ISBN: 978-1-78817-984-3
Audiobook ISBN: 978-1-78817-985-0

Interior illustrations: Lisa Lister

10 9 8 7 6 5 4 3 2 1

Printed in the United States of America

This product uses responsibly sourced papers and/or recycled
materials. For more information, see www.hayhouse.com.

*In dedication and devotion to the goddess Hathor,
the power and creativity of Ayvenuzijha, and
the Wild Roses, past, present, and future.*

Who trust and lead with their big and beauty-full hearts.

*Who choose, above all things, to Vivre La Vie
Vénusienne (Live the Venus Life), because EVERYTHING
sounds more delicious in French, doesn't it?*

Contents

Contents

IN THE KEY OF VENUS

SHE whispers, 'Enough. Stop.'

I stop.

I stop looking,

seeking

perfection in all things and sigh.

A big sigh.

SHE whispers, 'Your body knows how.'

I let go.

I let my body show me how natural it is to surrender.

My body, slowed all. the. way. down, falls deep.

Deep into the void.

Of NO thing.

The ancestors of the ancient-future come
to check my pulse in dreamtime.

They stay.

We circle and hum and sing remembered
magic, together, in the darkness.

Until I remember MY song.

MY note.

MY magic.

SHE whispers, 'It's in the key of Venus.'

The harmonics of the process.

Of the unfolding.

Of the unfurling.

Of the beauty.

Of the dreaming into reality, into human-ness.

Into the real and truth-y flesh and
bones of a life, fully lived.

Introduction

Venus.

A planet.

The ancient Roman goddess of love, sex, and beauty.

A term used to describe the small female figurines sculpted during the Upper Paleolithic Period (the early Stone Age) that are believed to be associated with fertility and sexuality.

A sugary sweet, heavily marketed version of pop culture femininity (mainly used to package and sell 'beauty' products to women).

AND… She's so much more.

She's astrological.

Cosmological.

Oracular.

Magnetic.

Mythical.

Mystical.

Cyclical.

Deeply feminine.

A path.

A frequency.

A sensual love affair with ALL of life.

This book is an invitation to journey with and embody all of Venus. To reconnect with and reclaim a lost lineage of knowing that brings together the energetic and the physical, the spiritual and the material, the Venus who has played a role in every culture since ancient times.

Everyone has a version of Venus, a goddess and a mythos attached to her; among the best known are Inanna, Ishtar, Freya, and Aphrodite. Yet some of my favorite women throughout time and space – from Mary Magdalene to Eleanor of Aquitaine, from Hathor to Sophia, from Joan of Arc to Anne Boleyn, and from the Atlantean queen Ash-ta-tara to Parisian literary queens Natalie Clifford Barney and Anaïs Nin – ALL knew/know the power that's held in the frequency of Venus.

Yes, the planet Venus's path in the sky has been mapped and tracked for millennia for both way-showing and guidance. Yet you need only look at the rhythmic cosmic dance in which Venus, Earth, and the sun participate to create the sacred geometry of the five-pointed pentagram AND the Wild Rose during Venus's eight-year cycle of death and rebirth to know that she also holds potent Divine Feminine wisdom and codes of power, creation, and love.

It's the frequency of Venus that we witness when we each express and show up in direct and harmonic relationship with our hearts. When we dare to share what it is that our hearts truly long for and desire, without apology. It's the acts of love we show to ourselves, to each other. It's how we adorn and decorate ourselves and the spaces and places we create and live in. It's our aesthetics, our magnetism, our values, our worth. It's the choice we make when we connect with the heart of another. It's Venus, embodied.

Which is why, in a world that feels like it's burning, in a world where making art and love and poetry and beauty have been made to seem superfluous, I've filled my favorite fountain pen with rose-scented ink and I'm offering my words, my art, as a love letter… to OUR hearts.

To the things that our hearts love.

To the daily acts of love that we make and create.

In devotion to Venus, the *wildest* of roses.

Why? Let me remind you…

Throughout time, temples have been dedicated to Venus and her mysteries and yet those temples have been desecrated or destroyed and the mysteries have been hidden. Patriarchal religions have deemed the temple practices – dance, ritual, art, music, nourishment, chanting, sacred sexuality, initiation, a knowledge of the sky, the stars, and the cosmos – frivolous, occultist, distracting, even sinister (remembering that the word 'sinister' refers to 'left-handed magic': the magic of the Divine Feminine.) Of COURSE they bloody have.

Loves, THIS is what we're here for.

To remember, reconnect with, reclaim, and revere ALL the things that have been called frivolous, distracting, and sinister. ALL the magic and medicine of Venus and her mysteries. So that we

dance, sing, ritualize, nourish, and Self Source ourselves, and each other, back to life.

Back to magic.

Back to power.

Back to love.

Back to Venus.

About this book

This book isn't just a transmission, it's also an affirmation and an activation. Because, let me be clear, to reconnect with, remember, reclaim, and revere Venus and her mysteries as a sacred path, a feminine frequency, and a sensual love affair with ALL of life is a defiant and really bloody necessary act of resistance in these wild and shifting times.

Defiant because it's energetic healing guided by our own inner authority. *Necessary* because when we become an embodied experience of the Venus frequency we have the capacity to make different choices; we use discernment, and we lead with love.

NOTE: Throughout the book, I refer to Venus as 'her/she' because that's the relationship I have with her. Ultimately, I believe that Venus represents the feminine principle/nature/ wisdom in each of us, regardless of gender, sexual orientation, or how you/I/we choose to identify on the glorious spectrum of being a human.

Venus is an initiator to creative feminine wisdom THROUGH our bodies, our beliefs, our sense of worth, because in an age of 'information overload,' it's the wisdom – feminine, intuited, felt, remembered, and experienced – that will nourish, satiate, and support us the most. It's how, amid the chaos of dying systems and structures, we can and will align and harmonize, root and magnetize, source and sustain to become the active Source-resses and Creatrixes of What. Comes. Next.

This book is a devotional, too. It's for each of us who:

* long to have our temple back. For community, for like-heartedness

* find remembering the magic and power in our bodies intense and overwhelming

* experience physical pain/discomfort at the idea of being 'seen' and 'known'

* have been told that our heart, and all that it desires, is NOT sacred and holy

* believe that our magic and our medicine, our power, as love, is 'frivolous' and 'unimportant'

* have forgotten that we're both divine AND a magnetic, creative force (and who can blame us? The societal spell is STRONG.) And that what we create – human life, a home, a business, art, peace in our bodies and being, or any of the gazillion other possibilities of which we're SO capable – matters.

Essentially, this book is the one that *I* would have LOVED to have read back when I was trying so desperately to connect the dots and make all that I was experiencing this lifetime – as a witch, a mystic, a creative, a lover, an artist, an oracle, and a woman – 'make sense.' *Spoiler alert:* It was ALL Venus. *Wink.*

I can't promise that I'll make everything 'make sense' to you. In fact, I KNOW I won't because that's NOT the point. However, I will help you to remember *why* you might experience challenge and resistance to life-living, magic, art, beauty, power, and love and introduce you to a lineage and legacy that I call the Wild Rose, which wants to support us as we re-tell and re-spell a new story.

Yes, I hold Venus keys and codes, and you do too. So, as is the case with everything I create, let a word, a phrase, an offering activate YOUR remembrance and YOUR wisdom. This isn't an astrology book, although I *will* talk about Venus as an astrological planet because knowing your astrological Venus placement (more on this coming up) can provide foundational wisdom and understanding about how to be in relationship with yourself and others and how to navigate WITH your heart.

And I'll also share ALL about the Venus cycle because it's something I've been tracking and mapping and sharing, both personally and in my online community, the SHE Power Collective, for many years and it's changed EVERYTHING for me.

NOTE: At this point, I want to say that the Venus cycle doesn't fit 'neatly' into our current calendars and clocks – it holds the feminine principle and opens the hidden mysteries of all of mother-loving creation, so of course it isn't bloody straightforward! But when you know where, and what, to pay attention to, it definitely becomes possible to attune with it.

Our Wild Rose path

When YOU come into alignment with Venus and her cycle you gain access to the super practical *and* very mystical Venusian magic and medicine that was dismissed and hidden from us so that we'd 'forget' how to cultivate, harness, and hold our feminine magic, medicine, power, and wisdom.

But what Venus and her Wild Rose lineage has returned *me* to, time and time again, is that the body *is* the mystery school. Bringing her esoteric and mystical teachings into fleshy reality THROUGH the body has been my most *powerful* Venus revealment. I call this the Wild Rose path and I've self-cultivated and curated it in direct relationship with Wild Roses throughout time and space (I meet with them in a Parisian-style salon in dreamtime – it's glorious, and I can't wait to introduce you to it and them.) AND my big, beauty-full, beat-y heart.

It's a remembered mystery school that's felt and sensed and forever revealing itself THROUGH my body. THROUGH my heart and all that it longs for and desires. THROUGH deep remembrance. THROUGH nature, the cosmos, and her divine, rhythmic intelligence.

It's how and why, in these wild and shifting times when we're told daily what we 'should' fear and hate, I choose to re-tell and re-spell my story:

* ❋ I'm a Self Source-ress who prioritizes my body, health, pleasure, and joy. A witch who can harness and hold my magic and power without depletion and/or burnout.

* ❋ I'm a lover of life who lets my heart lead. (And believe me, it takes me on the wildest adventures – usually to France, the place where my heart is always at its biggest. It's where this book was written because France is my lover. It's OK, my husband knows ALL about it; in fact, he often participates. *Wink.*)

❋ I'm an active Creatrix and collaborator of What. Comes. Next. An artist who paints hope and dreams and possibility in glorious technicolor. Not because I'm avoiding or afraid of the dark. No, I'm rooted in it. That's how I grow. That's how I THRIVE.

I want this for you too – or at least YOUR version of it – so I'll offer Venus's astrological symbol, often called a 'mirror,' as a key to unlock her whispers and mysteries reflected within *you*. Because gaining mistress-ry of Venus is to become the mistress of ALL of life. Together, we'll explore *all* the ways to prepare our bodies and nervous systems to 'hold' our magic, so that we're able to be seen, heard, and known.

No more hiding. Make out with every possibility and opportunity; seduce and be seduced by life; re-spell, re-enchant, and romance your entire life in the wisdom and bones and belly-deep knowing that Venus is love, art, creation, expansion, and beauty. And Venus is ALSO death and destruction, constriction, and grief. AND it's the entire life-lived spectrum of experience that sits in the space between. ALL. AT. THE. SAME. TIME.

Back to Venus

So yes, in this book, I'll share about the planet Venus, her mythos, her cycle and phases, the feminine frequency she holds. But mostly, I'm an enthusiast, a creative, a lover of all that Venus is and represents, and while you'll find countless books/ resources offering 'information' about Venus, what I share here is a love letter from my heart to yours. A felt experience.

It's *my* Wild Rose path. *My* connection to a lineage of Wild Roses, women – real, historical, archetypal, and mythic. An act of love in devotion to ALL things Venus, shared with you so that you too can create and explore YOUR Wild Rose path, direct from your heart, because:

Loves, THIS is what we're here for.

To remember, reconnect with, reclaim, and revere ALL the things that have been called frivolous, distracting, and sinister. ALL the magic and medicine of Venus and her mysteries. So that we dance, sing, ritualize, nourish, and Self Source ourselves, and each other, back to life.

Back to magic.

Back to power.

Back to love.

Back to Venus.

Beautiful and resilient, strong but with a delicate flower, the Wild Rose is often referred to as a 'weed' because it's untamable and grows in places and spaces where people would 'prefer' it didn't. In fact, Wild Roses blossom and bloom on their own terms and it's in the wildest of times here on planet Earth that I invite you/us to take our Venusian mirror, meet our gaze in its reflection, and declare ourselves Wild Roses.

WE ARE THE WILD ROSES.

We are *not* to be tamed.

Despite all the attempts to bury us, to make our landscape inhospitable and barren, to disconnect us from our roots, WE RETURN.

Still we bloom and still we thrive.

We are the Wild Roses who KNOW that our power is love.

Thank you for being here, Wild Rose.

BIG love to your beauty-full, beat-y, courageous heart. It is where entire revolutions can and *will* start.

Lisa x

Opening Ceremony

Welcome home. You've entered the most sacred of temple spaces. The sound of sistrums – the ancient Egyptian rattles associated with the Ma goddess Hathor – being shaken, along with a deep and rhythmic drumbeat, mark your entrance. (Yes, you're a big deal around here. You're seen, known, and loved, and everyone's been expecting you.)

You walk, barefoot, on a rose-petal-strewn path, and as you step, the petals release the most delicious, sweet perfume that combines with the frankincense incense and smoke sitting heavy in the air. You inhale deeply as you arrive at an altar draped in green silk, dedicated to Venus. Pink, green, and white candles are burning and there are delectable, juicy figs and pomegranate seeds, large pieces of rose quartz and collected shells, a loved-in journal and a pen filled with rose-scented red ink, and beautifully ornate jars holding rose, frankincense, and jasmine oil next to a cup of warm blue-lotus and rose-petal tea.

You pick your favorite of the three scents and anoint your third eye, your throat, your heart, and just below your belly button with dabs of oil. You open the journal to a clean page, take a bite from the juiciest fig, and when you finish savoring its fleshy goodness, with intention, you slowly sip the rose and blue-lotus tea. When you've drunk every drop, you say out loud:

Wild Roses, ancestors of this lineage, past, present, and future, throughout time, place, and space, we chant your names.

Hathor. Inanna. Cleopatra. Madonna. Mary Magdalene. Isis. Joan Jett. Aphrodite. Anaïs Nin. Madeleine de Scudéry. Sappho. Natalie Clifford Barney. Frida Kahlo. Anne Boleyn. Joan of Arc. Miley Cyrus. Dolly Parton. Lana Del Ray. (Add the names of the Wild Roses who speak to and through you.)

At the center of the altar is a mirror, set in a copper frame in the shape of the astrological symbol for Venus. You pick it up and you see that on the reverse is the sigil for the Wild Roses – *our* sigil, a cosmic wink throughout time and space to support *our* remembrance – and on the front, a simple, reflective surface.

You breathe deeply – in through the nose and out through the mouth – three times, audibly. You allow the breath to return to its usual place and pace in your body and let your body soften from the top all the way to the bottom. And then you look directly into the mirror and witness your reflection. You place a hand on your heart and meet yourself here, while you ask for direct counsel from and connectivity with Venus:

Venus, SHE of beauty, harmonics, sensual pleasure, and creative vision, I call to you. I am open to receive and ready to remember, reconnect with, reclaim, and revere the Venusian mysteries THROUGH my body.

You keep breathing deeply as a white light with rose-pink sparkling particles comes down, through the top of your head, through your throat, into your heart, and down into your pelvic bowl. Hold that pink sparkling light in that space, in your pelvic bowl, your medicine bowl, as a white light with pink sparkling particles comes up from the core of Mumma

Earth – through your cervix, your root – and meets the pink sparkling light already in your pelvic bowl. The light from above meeting the light from below, IN YOUR BODY.

You recognize the rose-pink sparkling light in your pelvic bowl, pull it up to your heart space, and ask for the Venus emerald-green ray of the heart to be activated:

I activate the Venus emerald-green ray of the heart.

You feel, sense, and witness any and all sensations that this emerald-green light of the heart may be creating in you, and you say:

Venus, I am open to receive.

You breathe in deeply, release a deep sigh, and let yourself be open to Venus speaking to and through you. It may be words, sensations, names, feelings, emotions, colors, textures, tastes, images, faces, and places – Venus has access to ALL of your sensorial nature. You're here for as long as feels good. Make notes, draw any images or codes that may make themselves known to you in this space. Allow your body to be a receiver, a divination rod of Venusian energetics – keys, codes, and symbols and teachings of feminine wisdom – and let them reveal themselves to you, THROUGH you.

A self-initiation occurs when you come into direct relationship with Venus. When you realize and recognize that your body is remembering and awake to the Venus Mystery School. The Mystery School that becomes fully realized through acts of love, ritual, dance, beauty, devotion, song, poetry, art, and nourishment for ALL THOSE who are prepared to develop the capacity to hold, hear, feel, and receive it. You say:

I (insert your name) am a Wild Rose and my body is a Venus Mystery School.

The Wild Roses are many, and our lineage is strong. We've been hiding in plain sight throughout lifetimes and time lines, our magic and mysteries encoded through art, myth, dance, and song. We've been called by many names – witches, healers, harlots, queens, and noblewomen – and we KNOW that Venus has no ONE truth: She offers many different fractals, different ways of perceiving her, in relation to her place in space and time.

As you feel your time in the temple come to an end, you meet your gaze in the mirror and say:

I commit to remember, reconnect with, reclaim, and revere ALL the things that have been called frivolous, distracting, and sinister. ALL the magic and medicine of Venus and her mysteries. So that we dance, sing, ritualize, nourish, and Self Source ourselves, and each other, back to life.

Back to magic.

Back to power.

Back to love.

You bow in reverence to Venus, bow in reverence to the Wild Roses – both ancient and future. And you bow to yourself as a Venus Mystery School, your body as life, magic, power, and love.

AND SO IT MOTHER-LOVING IS.

NOTE: You can re-create this ritual for yourself or simply let it be an imaginal experience of re-enchantment that unfurls in your being as you read it. (I'm a ceremonialist, so I get a little 'extra' when it comes to creating ceremony and ritual. Also, Friday is a Venus day, so if you *are* called, making time and space to connect with her on a Friday is ALWAYS a good idea.)

Venus Correspondences

Correspondences are a list of things that, well, correspond with and are associated with the energetics of a particular thing; in our case, Venus. You can use one, several, or all of the correspondences below to connect with, meditate on, create, and make your own Venusian magic and medicine.

Day: Friday.

Astrological signs that She rules: Taurus and Libra.

Venus in Her power: Love. Fertility. Attraction. Resources. Money. Romance. Beauty. Aesthetics. Magnetism. Harmony. Pleasure. Relationships. Sensuality. Luxury. Desire. Sexuality. Values. Worth. Ease. Joy. Art. Fashion. Social life. Charm. Intuition.

Venus Hotspots: Overindulgence. Vanity. Debauchery. Illusion. Addiction.

Animals: Doves. Swans.

Deities: Inanna and Ishtar (Mesopotamian); Venus (Roman); Aphrodite (Greek); Freya (northern European); Lakshmi and Lalita Devi (Hindu).

Plants and herbs: Roses. Peonies. Mugwort. Myrtle. Blue lotus. Damiana. Jasmine. Benzoin. Violets. Tonka. Hibiscus. (I combine rose, blue lotus, damiana, jasmine, and hibiscus to make teas to drink and bathe in – SO Venusian!)

Food: Figs. Dates. Pomegranates. Honey. Cacao. Vanilla. Sweet fruits such as mangoes, raspberries, and strawberries. (To be honest, I believe ANYTHING that tastes delicious, succulent, juicy, ripe, and decadent can, and *should*, be considered Venusian!)

Crystals and minerals: Rose quartz. Emerald. Copper. Coral. Turquoise. Lodestone. Peridotite. Cobaltoan Calcite, also known as Aphrodite stone (I wear an Aphrodite stone on my Venus finger – the third finger. On the left hand, it's the one on which you might wear a wedding ring.)

Colors: Pink. Green. Rose gold.

Tarot card associations: The Empress. The Two of Cups (love). The Nine of Disks (gain).

Magic work with Venus: Friday is a great day for self-love practices, romantic dates, building relationships, buying yourself flowers, and tending to yourself with ALL the love.

Venus energy is essentially stored solar energy, so you can use its 'stored potential' to build your resources and prosperity. We'll be talking more about the astrology of Venus later, but when the sun is in the Earth sign of Taurus, you can work with Venus to call in and create material wealth and physical pleasure, tend to the relationship that you have with your self, and connect with your sensuality through your body and senses.

And when the sun is in the Air sign of Libra, you can work with Venus to call in and create lasting and powerful relationships with others – both platonic and romantic – and assess your values and acknowledge your worth so that you're able to direct your own value and worth in the world.

Other Venus-related things to know: Venus is the second planet from the sun and she's the third brightest object in the sky after the sun and moon. She goes her own way, literally: She rotates slowly in the opposite direction to most other planets. (She's contrary, and we LOVE that about her.)

April 1 is Veneralia, an ancient Roman festival of Venus. It's said that worshippers would drape statues of the goddess with wreaths of myrtle (which we love) to venerate her and to call in good fortune (which we also love). And also, to help the hearts (and vulvas) of girls and women to be, and to remain, 'pure' and 'chaste' (basically, what I perceive as an attempt to control women and their sexuality, which we absolutely do NOT love.)

This is why I've reclaimed Veneralia and renamed it the Day of the Wild Roses – OUR DAY. I actively encourage us ALL to circle April 1 in the diary and defiantly, with ALL the love, buy ourselves flowers, chocolates, a gift to celebrate ourselves as women; to self-pleasure, to have amazing sex, to orgasm LOTS (and on our terms) in DEVOTION to ourselves, to pleasure, to our bodies, to Venus.

NOTE: How you choose to work with any of this is YOUR call and your responsibility. Please use fierce self-care when using herbs and oils specifically: Check for allergies, and whether they're safe if you're pregnant or experiencing health issues that they may exacerbate.

Venus:
Who Is She?

Planet, myth, archetype, muse, marketing concept – Venus is *many* things. When I was five years old my mumma introduced me to Venus in her morning and evening star phases in the sky, and I've been captivated ever since by her ability to be more than one possibility.

In fact, it's my fascination with Venus *as* Ma, as creative force – an all-encompassing representation of SHE as Creatrix – that's led me on the wildest of SHE quests and adventures around the world as I've sought out and experienced what are known as Venus figures. These mostly small statuettes of females with large breasts, hips, and bums (and some with exposed vulvas) were created during the Upper Paleolithic Period (which lasted from about 50,000–40,000 years ago until around 10,000 years ago), although similar stylized representations of women were produced in the period that followed, the Neolithic.

The most famous of these female icons is the Venus of Willendorf, who was carved from limestone more than 27,000 years ago. She was discovered in Austria in 1908 and can be seen today in Vienna's Natural History Museum; when they first unearthed her, she was fully covered in red ochre, which an archaeologist accidentally rubbed off. Now

Austria's best-known archaeological find, she was/is indicative of a culture that worshipped women and mothers as life-givers and goddesses. (I wear a silver ring with a likeness of the Venus of Willendorf in celebration of chubby woman mumma goodness!)

The discovery of prehistoric Venus figures, along with other finds in temple complexes such as those in Malta, one of my most favorite SHE locales, points to the existence of early matrifocal societies. And this is where the Venus 'story' gets *really* interesting to me, because these representations pre-date the Roman goddess Venus by *thousands* of years. More than 250 of them have been excavated in the last century, at sites ranging from the Pyrenees to Siberia, suggesting there were once peaceful women- and goddess-centered civilizations represented by 'Venus.'

NOTE: Using the word 'Venus' to describe these ancient female icons has been hotly debated in recent years, with many calling it a degrading and diminishing term for something that's so powerful and important. I get it. AND I strongly believe that WE get to place our power back into the terms and words that are used against us or in a derogatory way. The words witch, hag, cunt, and pythoness, for example, have been used to demean women, yet we've reclaimed them by breathing our power and truth back into them and saying them out loud as our own. And I very much feel that we're doing the same here and now with Venus.

Venus through time and space

Now, when we chart the different 'versions' of Venus and her mythos across time it's very clear to me that she's something of a shape-shifter, becoming what's 'necessary' for the age in which she finds herself. Some would say that this was done *to* her, and I'd agree that in some periods there was a distinct objective to distort, defame, and devalue both Venus and the Mother – to actively detach us from her. AND YET... Venus as the feminine frequency, the Wild Rose, ALWAYS finds a way.

As all myths and stories do, the 'Venus mythos' has changed as the societies in which her story is told have changed – from the early Mesopotamian and Egyptian tales of Inanna, Ishtar, and Hathor to those of the later Greek and Norse Persephone and Freya. And that's just in North Africa, Europe, and southwest Asia; in India, the goddess Durga has evolved over time into her own Venusian aspects: Lakshmi and Lalita Devi. In fact, all world cultures have an archetypal version of Venus because she IS the feminine frequency. And I feel that all the versions of Venusian deity-fication carry the frequency of the Divine Feminine.

SHE.

Ma.

Creatrix of all alchemizing divinity to matter.

Matter to divinity.

Over and over.

It's the nature of ALL creation.

The descent.

The path IN to NO thing.

The void.

NO thing from which EVERY thing is possible.

Pure potentiality.

From which ALL things can then rise.

The womb. The cosmic womb.

The Mumma. The cosmic Mumma.

The divine nature of the feminine.

Now, I believe it's THIS remembrance that they're most afraid of. It's WHY there's been a conscious desire to disconnect us (and maintain that disconnection) from the worship of Ma and take the power practices associated with it – feminine magic, sensuality, sound currents, ecstatic dance, discernment, persuasion, magnetism, and manifestation – and use them outside of the container of love, compassion, and devotion for personal gain.

Look, the myths and stories of post-matrifocal civilizations were largely populated by heroes and war disciples so that the people would serve a ruler and be controllable and willing to fight for their 'empire.' Tales of creation, love, nurture, and care were/are few and far between because it's much harder to manipulate and control those who have faith and trust in Ma, as Creatrix. Those who witness *themselves* as Ma, Creatrix.

The Venus mythos

What I share here are light-touch summaries of some of the key stories and myths we've been told in relation to the archetypal image of Venus. I've found that we often become 'needy' for comprehensive and/or scholarly understanding, but you won't find that here. As with everything I write and share, the invitation is to soften and receive, to tune in to your heart and deeper knowing and then *feel* what's being said and what's *not* being said.

As you read about these Venus archetypes/stories, you *might* feel that one of them speaks louder to you than the others. Whether this happens is dependent on many things, among them your upbringing and your societal, familial, cultural, and religious beliefs. For example, the Venus archetype Inanna feels fleshy and real to *me*, while Aphrodite… not so much.

That's the beauty, *literally*, of Venus's shape-shifting nature – as a feminine frequency throughout time and space, she's remained 'available' and relevant to every one of us who is fertile and fecund ground to receive and hold her frequency.

Here's a time line of the Venus mythos:

* **Inanna/Ishtar** – 3,200–331 BCE, Mesopotamia, southwest Asia
* **Hathor/Isis** – c.3,000 BCE–332 CE, Egypt
* **Persephone/Aphrodite/Venus** – c.1200 BCE–c.500 CE, Greece and Rome
* **Mary Magdalene** – 1st century CE, Palestine, eastern Mediterranean
* **Freya** – c.700 CE, northern Europe

Inanna/Ishtar

The earliest story of 'Venus,' and my personal favorite, is that of the descent to the underworld of Inanna, a popular goddess in the mythology of the Sumerians of Mesopotamia (an area that today forms part of Iraq and Syria); later Mesopotamian peoples, the Babylonians and Assyrians, called her Ishtar. We'll be 'myth mapping' this tale later in the book as it's one of the first known interpretations of the planetary movement of Venus from morning star to evening star, depicting both descent and ascent, night and day, light and dark, death and rebirth.

Hathor/Isis

Hathor, the Egyptian Ma goddess who's often depicted wearing a headdress of cow horns with a solar disk between them, was regarded as THE goddess, from whom all other goddesses originated. Hathor's associated with women's health – some suggest that the image of her face on the walls of Egypt's Dendera temple represents the female reproductive system – as well as mummahood, fertility, joy, celebration, music, dance, and the afterlife. She's also often referred to as the mumma of civilization. No Big Deal.

Now, back in the day in Egypt, the high priestess to Hathor was also the queen, and she was absolutely seen and revered as an extension of the goddess and her power. She too became the Great Mother love. She too was a Creatrix, and she ensured harmony between people, nature, and source power, all in Hathor's name.

Temples, also in Hathor's name, were dedicated to the planetary movements of the sun and Venus, with their cycles a metaphor for moving through the cyclical death, rebirth, and rejuvenation processes required for us all to experience ourselves as divine, self-realized, creative power and magic.

Hathor's traits and characteristics, including her solar disk, were later absorbed into those of the goddess Isis (one of the most important Egyptian deities). It's within this lineage, it's said, that Mary Magdalene herself was a high initiate, and when I remember, reconnect with, reclaim, and revere the Venusian mysteries through MY own body as a mystery school, THIS is what I continually return to.

Birthing, sustaining, refining, and aligning, moving through the cyclical death, rebirth, and rejuvenation processes, over and over, to remember ourselves as divine, self-realized, creative power and magic. Hathor magic. Venus magic. OUR magic.

I will forever shake my sistrum – the ancient rattle said to ward off evil, inspire goodness, and open portals – in love and reverence to Hathor. In fact, I'm weaving this entire book under the starry gaze and guidance of the goddess Hathor because I believe she is THE Wild Rose. Our rooted wisdom. Our all-the-way-back medicine keeper of the Ma frequency, of the Venusian mysteries; to what it is we KNOW and are remembering (and need to keep remembering) to create a new possibility here on Earth.

Persephone

The most important myth about the ancient Greek goddess Persephone reveals an evolution from the hunter-gatherer/ agrarian societies of ancient Mesopotamia to the 'war-led' societies of ancient Greece and Rome. While Inanna enters the underworld *knowingly*, Persephone, daughter of Zeus, the chief god, and Demeter, goddess of agriculture, is abducted by Hades, king of the underworld, and taken there against her will. She 'marries'/loses her innocence to Hades, who 'tricks' her into eating the 'forbidden fruit' – oh, where have we heard that before?

The fruit is a pomegranate, an ancient representation of life, fertility, and regeneration, and as a consequence of eating the seeds of the pomegranate, Persephone must spend six months of the year in the underworld with Hades and six months of the year with her mother in the upper world. We witness the pain and loss that Demeter feels at being separated from her daughter: During the months of the year that Persephone is away from her, the goddess causes Earth to wither and die, which to the Greeks explained autumn and winter. And the six months in which Persephone is released and reunited with her mother signal the renewal of hope, new beginnings, and the fertility of the lands – or spring and summer.

As human civilizations became more complex and sophisticated, the Venusian stories evolved in order to fit the needs and requirements of the societies they represented. As we move to the myths of Aphrodite and Venus as Greek/Roman goddesses, we recognize that they are similar in nature. And when myths and stories came from Africa into Europe, they were, for want of a better term, 'patriarch-ed' by the institutions and culture of the time to fit *their* own needs and requirements.

Aphrodite/Venus

In ancient Greece, Aphrodite was worshipped as a goddess of the sea and seafaring, but she was mainly associated with love, beauty, sexual desire, and pleasure. Later, the Romans adopted Aphrodite's mythos, symbols, and characteristics for their goddess Venus. Eventually she was distilled to the two very basic archetypes of love and lust – virgin and whore – and her only REAL job was to sire heroes for the new war myths, look 'pretty,' and 'fuck the war' out of men/soldiers before they returned home to their families. (This was in fact a sacred act of sexuality performed by temple priestesses that was later distorted and called 'prostitution.')

There are two versions of the origin story of Aphrodite/Venus. The first gives her a marine birth: When the Titan (or giant) Cronos severed his father Uranus's genitals and threw them in the sea, the blood and semen caused a white foam to form and come to the land of Cyprus. It was there that a naked Venus rose from the sea out of the foam – as depicted by Sandro Botticelli in his famous 1485 painting 'The Birth of Venus.'

The other version, told by the Greek poet Homer, has Aphrodite/Venus as the daughter of Zeus and the ocean nymph Dione. In this story, she married Hephaestus, god of fire and the forge, and had children. Venus wasn't interested in domestic duties (same girl, same) and was much more invested in matters of the heart – love and lust – among the gods and mortals.

Aphrodite/Venus had many loves, including the god Mars (Aries) and the mortal Adonis. She was also the mother of Cupid, the Roman god of love, and Deimos and Phobos, the Greek gods of fear and dread. (I mean, if we're looking to demonize the mumma, make her responsible for birthing love *and* fear *and* dread. Just saying.)

NOTE: With Aphrodite/Venus we witness the sea connection – the Mer lineage: the remembrance that ALL life evolved from the sea. Every organism in our ecosystem responds to, and is biologically linked through, water. We live in the embryological fluid of our mumma's womb for nine months, so living in water is a core, cellular memory for us. We're from the sea, we are the sea. We carry the learnings and yearnings of our oceanic ancestors IN our bodies. And for me, this is Venus.

The Marys

In Christianity, while SHE may not have a starring role, Mumma Mary was/is ever-present. And I'm pretty sure you already know that Mary Magdalene was demoted, defamed, and her story *heavily* distorted, despite the fact she was Jesus's consort and very definitely Main Character Energy. Yet Mary, in ALL her forms – virgin, mumma, whore, Black – remains. They are ALL Venus as a feminine frequency because the Wild Rose *always* finds a way.

NOTE: I'm often asked what's with my fascination for religious sites and the stories of religious women. Especially since religious institutions have a 'sketchy' (at best) record when it comes to treating and representing women well.

My response? You'll have seen and recognized in the last few years how easily and quickly certain views and opinions that disagree with the mainstream narrative are shut down and censored. So, in order to share the feminine frequency, Venus – the thread that holds the real and true magic and medicine of the feminine through the ages (especially in times when it wasn't safe for us to share our medicine and magic) – sometimes, a more 'pleasing to the mainstream' narrative must be told/provided.

In this way, the frequency can continue to exist for times, like now, when those of us with 'eyes to see' can read 'between' what's said and not said; what's been coded for us to unlock and remember THROUGH our body, because that's OUR magic.

When I lived in Malta – the islands I was called to because of their 5,000+ year-old temples where many Venus figurines have been and continue to be discovered – I saw that roads are named after Mumma Mary and there are shrines to her on every street corner. In the village I lived in, I'd watch the women go to pray to her in the morning and the evening when the church bells would call. I'd give EVERY shrine a knowing wink (and sometimes she'd wink right back at me), because I believe to worship Her is to worship Venus, the Divine Feminine frequency, love, in each and every one of us.

Freya

As Christianity spread throughout and beyond the Roman Empire, it really doubled down on the 'one male god' idea, the 'demonization' of the Divine Feminine, and removing the 'need' for feminine gods and their mythos entirely. Don't get me started on THAT. However, in the lands of northern Europe, the pagan gods and traditions persisted – hurrah. This was largely because their rugged terrain made it hard for the invading armies to reach them. Which meant that Freya, the Nordic version of Venus, 'survived' for a long time after the advent of Christianity.

Freya was/is known as a queen, a mother, a witch, a warrior, a 'noble' incarnation of feminine power; she has many 'handmaids' who represent the various facets and aspects of her nature. It took until the 12th century for Christians to convert the pagan northern and Slavic tribes to their faith, and even then, they had mixed success.

It takes time for ideas and thoughts to spread and take root, and in some parts of the world Christian missionaries were unable to convert the entire population to their faith. In India, for example, in the very powerful polytheistic religion of Hinduism we still witness Venus in the goddesses Lakshmi, Saraswati, Parvati, and even Lalita Devi – the many facets of the feminine frequency expressed in a way that's meaningful to those who are receiving her.

The mirror of Venus

On a recent visit to northern France, I sat with a very beautiful Black Madonna statue. Black Madonnas are a BIG part of my own Gypsy/Traveller tradition, with the most famous being the one that represents Sara-la-Kali, queen/saint of the Gypsies,

Romani, and Travellers, in the village of Saintes-Maries-de-la-Mer in southern France.

These mystical Black Madonnas, which I believe are SUPER esoteric, are found in fully 'religious' sites; and remember, anywhere they've built a church, you can guarantee it's sat above a potent and sacred magic power point and what that represents. The Black Madonna, specifically, is *very* heavily associated with Venus and the rose paths, and to Magdalene Medicine and magic: the feminine magic of Venus that was kept by many secret societies throughout time and space, including European priestesses, queens, and noble types (many in France) who guarded the Divine Feminine mysteries during the medieval period. It's ALL CONNECTED.

As I sat with this Black Madonna, I lit a candle to her and petitioned her. I wrote her a love note. This is my 'thing' in sacred sites; I'll always open my notebook and ask for whoever I'm in conversation with to write through me. (It's a good practice, and I recommend it.) This is what she shared:

You've written words, shared practices, given people instructions and maps to explore their bodies and their power and their magic. Good. Now you need to go deeper. Yes, you've come in and come down. Now come in FURTHER, come down DEEPER. Shit is going to get VERY real, VERY human. AND it's going to get as divine AS FUCK.

Call in the WILD ROSES. Remember Venus as a sacred path, a feminine frequency, a sensual love affair with life. Follow YOUR rose line. Say yes to YOUR magic. Say yes to life and love. Say yes to you as the mother-loving mystery school. Human AND divine. WHOLE and HOLY. WHOLY.

This wasn't the first time I'd heard this message; in fact, the most significant occasion prompted me to write this book. I was in Paris on my astrological Venus Return and tracing Venus's rose lines there – the city holds *many* keys and codes for those of us who identify with a rose path; the rose is the official flower of Paris, and the feminine frequency of Venus is literally in her waters and begins at the 'source.' *Wink.* I was told by SHE (because HER voice is REALLY loud there): 'Follow your rose line,' with the emphasis on *your*.

Now, hearing those words raised *far* more questions than answers, as is so often the case when we work with the feminine frequency. But, as someone who LOVES astrology and specifically astrocartography (using our astrological natal/birth chart details to analyze and understand how and why specific places and locations in the world affect us), I took them quite literally. I started following *my* rose line, my astrological Venus line, which runs through many very potent and magical power points in France. Which is how I came to be sat at the feet of *this* particular Black Madonna.

Don't worry, this book is NOT solely about my personal explorations of my own Venus/rose line. (Although, quite frankly, that *would* be an amazing book. The STORIES! Not least the one where, on another trip to Paris, I collapsed in the street and SHE sent THREE of her hottest firemen – the pompiers of Paris are a THING! – to carry me like Cleo-freakin'-patra. It was scary, it was near-death-y, it was thrilling, and there was a rebirth – eventually, months later. And well, it was all SO very Venus.)

Feeling what's real

No, this book is about the re-telling and re-spelling of my story based on what's revealed itself in the mirror of Venus, through my own body as a living mystery school. That's now become *my* Venus myth, *my* rose path, my Wild Rose path, as I *vis la vie vénusienne* – live the Venusian life.

France, to me, is the most powerful Venusian teacher. She's taught me to romance myself because she romances me. She whispers, in the most glorious and seductive French accent: *If you continue to stay where love isn't, Lisa, the poetry? The art? The magic? It will die.* She shows me that what I choose to accept is what I ultimately get more of. So, I must *only* accept what I want more of. And I want... More love. More creativity. More magic. More art. More music. More dance. More ALIVENESS.

Venus very much represents our relationship to *all* things, so if we let it, and we absolutely *should* let it, the feminine frequency can redefine and realign our relationship with our bodies, with each other, with pleasure, joy, sex, money, beauty, receiving, abundance, rest... *everything*.

But we only ever feel what's real. I don't meet Venus through *ideas* of her; I meet her through conversations with other women, in the art I devour, in the words I read, the music I hear, the magic and the miracles I experience and keep choosing to experience. Which all encourage me to be *more* alive.

Who is Venus to you?

Look, I love a great myth, and among the many, many stories told about Venus throughout the ages there will no doubt be one or two that provoke and evoke certain memories and sensations in your body and being in the same way that those of Inanna, Hathor, Mary Magdalene, and the Black Madonna do for me. It's been fascinating for me to realize and recognize that the deity/goddess archetypes that I've been called to throughout *this* lifetime are ALL Women of the Wild Rose/Venus archetypes/ keepers of the Creatrix power of Ma, the feminine frequency.

And as I share in all my work, when it comes to the stories we're told – specifically those about women and their archetypal nature, from Pandora to Cassandra, and from Lilith to Eve – PLEASE get curious. So much of human history – in particular, HER story – has not been recorded in our favor. Sometimes it's not been recorded at all and has therefore been lost forever; which, while absolutely true, is also NOT true (because the feminine is NOTHING if not contrary, right?!) I say this because we DO have the capacity to remember. Yes, it's a skill, but it's one that we all have access to, specifically us as women. And to 'remember' and to 'know' in a world that's obsessed with information and proof is HOW we're going to cocreate What Comes Next. But we must *believe* that we can.

You don't need to be ready, but you DO need to be courageous.

Write your own Venus story

We've been *told* that Venus is both love and war.

We've been *told* that Venus is sugary sweet and a 'good girl.'

We've been *told* that Venus is sex and desire.

We've been *told*, through the depictions of her in male-made art, that Venus is a fair-skinned beauty who was birthed naked from the sea.

But the REAL question is:

What's YOUR Venus story?

Who is SHE and what does she represent to you?

I invite you to meditate and riff on these questions.

What ignites a flame of knowing in you? What feels off? What stories are missing? I've barely scratched the surface here in terms of the stories and cultures of Venus throughout time and space. Maybe your lineage and spiritual beliefs will lead you down a very different Venus path.

Come into YOUR body.

Come into YOUR heart and meet Venus there.

Take the enquiry into your dreamtime and witness what unfolds.

Remember what you FEEL and KNOW to be true. NOT what you've been told.

Let the many stories of Venus help you to remember YOUR unsung siren song. Your personal myth. You, as an ever-evolving, shape-shifting channel for creation. And write, experience, and most importantly, fully live, YOUR Venus story. One that, for a start, isn't written by a dude. One where you walk (talk, sing, and dance) a self-curated sacred path in service to the feminine frequency, Ma, source, creative force. YOUR Wild Rose path (and yes, you do get to, and absolutely *should*, throw your own mother-loving rose petals.)

And please, for the love of Cleopatra, Joan Jett, Mary Magdalene, and Dolly Parton, make it a story worth telling. Dare to make YOUR Venus story the most glorious, fun-filled, salacious, juicy, and delicious adventure anyone has ever heard/read/witnessed (and if there's a chance that it would be heavily censored or even banned in certain US states? Well, then you KNOW you're on the right track. *Wink.*)

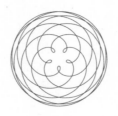

Magic, art, beauty, romance, and poetry are always available.

Life WANTS to romance you.

The Wild Rose

The Wild Rose is remembering and reclaiming and returning.

Curating and creating, reconstructing and reconsecrating the Venus mysteries.

Of the feminine.

Of Ma.

THROUGH YOU.

As we navigate these wild and shifting times here on Earth, the siren call is for us to come out of hiding and remember that WE are the ones who are going to create What Comes Next.

Now, I won't lie, I'm not entirely comfy making such big, bold statements. And I feel like it's THIS that many of us - especially those who identify as witches - are most worried about, because we've got *really* good at hiding and keeping secrets. We've had to; we've done it for entire lifetimes and across many, many time lines.

The sun (our identity, who we are) and Mumma Earth (the Great Ma, matter) are in cahoots with Venus (harmony, love, and beauty) and between them, in their delicious cosmic dance, they are calling the Wild Roses - that's us, BTW - to gather. Yep, ALL who have hidden and kept secrets *sub rosa* ('under the rose') have birthed us over and over. We've birthed ourselves over and over, with the codes of Venus, so that we can now remember. We each hold a thread, the Venus keys and codes that will support ALL OF HUMANITY (no pressure) to realize and recognize who we really are – divine creative power and magic. And our fierce responsibility is to create harmony within ourselves and our bodies, with each other, with nature, and with the divine (which isn't easy when so many of us have been infantilized by societal programming).

SHE snakes through the half-forgotten and distorted stories. From the rose-petal-strewn, red-ochre path of Inanna to the Venus of Willendorf, who, it's said, was carved from stone carried from Lake Garda in Italy – the lady of the lake. The blood-red realization that all life comes from the water. Maybe there's something to the Aphrodite/Venus 'birth' story after all: a red-headed beauty – as she's depicted in Botticelli's painting 'The Birth of Venus' – rising from the sea. So many of the stories (as well as the art, architecture, archetypes, signs, and symbols) have meanings that are hiding in plain sight.

And as Wild Roses? Our magic is to weave, un-weave, and re-weave the mysteries – to re-tell and re-spell them for These Times.

Venus and the Wild Rose path

And it's THIS rose line, the mother line of the wildest rose, that moves through our bodies and our DNA. Ancient codes of priestesses and witches and healers and wise ones are activated when WE remember.

When we remember that we hold the vermilion red thread that runs directly from the heart of SHE who contains all life.

SHE who nurtures. SHE who has wild, passionate sex. SHE who descends. SHE who is Ma of the Dark Matter. SHE who eats the sun and births the moon. SHE who KNOWS the dark. Intimately. SHE who knows how to grow strong roots and rise, rebirth, and create a mother-loving renaissance. All of THIS is encoded in YOU.

LOVE. BEAUTY. MAGIC. HARMONY. LIBERATION. CREATION. POWER.

And we activate those codes when we commit to Venus. To the Wild Rose path. To remembered power and magic. Mysteries mistress-ed. A devotion to love as an alchemical force. To a passionate, sensual, and romantic love affair with our life.

NOTE: I'm *fully* aware that the idea of having a romantic love affair with life may feel like one of those thick, glossy coffee-table books that share ALL the ways in which its author is living this gorgeous, delicious, idyllic existence. In the soft-focus photos, she's wearing a floaty white dress that looks like a Victorian nightgown; a flaky croissant sits before her on a mismatched (on purpose) plate on a whimsical tablecloth, and she sips a steaming cup of just-poured-from-the-cafetière coffee.

As she gazes out the window at the raised vegetable beds she cultivates herself, a mid-morning shard of sunlight catches her in just the right way. And I won't lie, she looks REALLY smug as she tells us, 'If I can create this, so can you. It's so easy.'

Except it's not always, is it? Well, I can tell you one thing for SURE: It was almost impossible, according to *my* cynical side eye and Scorpio shade-thrower. Both of which, for most of my life, have acted as *the* most powerful defensive safety armor. Because the scariest thing I could ever do was to let *anything* be safe and easy. To let the beauty, art, and poetry of life romance and enchant the SHIT out of me over and over again. And for me to be in a sensual love affair with... well, ALL OF IT? FUCK, NO. NO. THANK. YOU.

Look, there are a gazillion reasons why this is the case for me – I come from a Traveller family, my parents got divorced, everyone I loved died within the space of 13 months, a boy I thought was my forever love went back on his word and left me to rebuild my life from scratch at my Saturn Return. If we need proof that life is to be feared and that people aren't trustworthy, I promise you we'll find it.

AND... if you want proof that life is really freaking beauty-full and magical and that people *can* be gorgeous and loving, you'll find that too. All that shitty stuff? It DID and DOES and WILL continue to happen. That's how being a human works. And my life IS magical. For sure, I've worked for it. AND... that doesn't stop it being really fucking magical. Because both can be true at the same time.

I've ALWAYS believed in magic. I've ALWAYS believed in love. But life, well... life can get very real life-y and those societal spells of fear, doubt, shame, and blame are REALLY BLOODY STRONG. Add to that the grief, the deaths (real and metaphorical), the disorientation, the let-downs, the heartbreak, the fear and horror, the very real urge to disassociate and numb out, and it's no wonder that I/you/we forget.

Although, I will say that how quickly we're able to 'catch ourselves' in the act is, for me at least, proof of how 'well' we're navigating and negotiating the human experience. And it makes *choosing* to stay present, to believe in love and magic, to fully be alive FOR life, a choice.

Connecting and working with Venus

This has been *my* most powerful Venus experiment and exploration: to choose, and to keep choosing, to return, and to keep returning to Venus and her mysteries, THROUGH my body and being, as an act of love and devotion. To let my body be the storyteller AND the mystery school. To recognize myself *as* a Wild Rose.

For me, working and connecting with Venus has REALLY supported the realizations and the revealments of what my deep feminine wisdom has *always* known – the fact that so much magic, art, beauty, romance, and poetry is always available; that life WANTS to romance me/you/us. Yet my stories – specifically those regarding my sense of worth and value, what I'm 'allowed' to have and how it must be 'worked' for – have kept me 'humble' and 'likeable.' And they've also kept me from truly enjoying, relishing, and devouring every deliciously heartbreaking, passionate, joyful, and pain-inducing bite of life.

The armor, which in my case came (and on occasion still does) predominantly in the shape of shade, sarcasm, and cynicism, has kept me from feeling and experiencing and living it ALL to the fullest. The need to please and appease means I've said yes when I meant to say no. I've curtailed and retreated and vowed never to shine brightly again. I've let what other people *might* say or think about me dictate the moves and direction I make and take. That was, until… I made a choice.

A choice to live as the **wildest** of roses.

To be re-enchanted by, and with, the WHOLE of life.

To have my hunger, my desires, satiated and to let joy ALL. THE. WAY. IN.

Y'see, Venus *really* wants us to LIVE. She wants us to be seen, to be courageous – to not be afraid of the material world but live a big, bold, and beauty-full life by activating our remembered magic: our feminine wisdom, our magnetic power, our capacity to create our destiny. And it feels VERY important and necessary to me to point out that 'activating our remembered magic' isn't going to be just a 'fun' thing we get to do in our spare time anymore. It will become an absolute necessity if we're to navigate the waves of These Times and play an active role in shaping What Comes Next.

I believe that our collective siren call is to believe in, and to be in service to, love.

Romantic love. Fierce love. Passionate love. Creative love. Compassionate love. Tender love.

(And a gazillion other words that YOU may associate with what it means to believe and to be in service to love.)

This will involve the following:

* Your heart being all-the-way open AND your boundaries strong.

* Your level of compassion (for ALL that's unfolding) being high AND your roots planted deep. (Into Ma of the Dark Matter.)

* Being ALL-SEEING (able to witness the terror, the horror, the war, the destruction AND the magic and the miracles. AT. THE. SAME TIME. AND having the capacity to get stretchy enough to hold them all without depletion or burnout.

* Creating and reshaping reality accordingly.

Becoming a Venusian Vessel

We KNOW that the current structures and systems are not, and never have been, set up in favor of supporting women and other humans who are remembering their magic. AND we KNOW that those structures and systems are most definitely in their final death-rattle phase – the timer is ticking, we can feel it and we can see it. And of course, THEY are not going down without a fight. And while THEY are NOT it, I am VERY much aware that those of us who are working in the realms of the feminine and flow DO NEED a container.

Our magic, medicine, and power NEED a place and space to return to as it's remembered.

Our magic, medicine, and power NEED to be held.

Our magic, medicine, and power NEED to be Self Source-ed so that we can integrate and potentize and alchemize. We let what we need grow in strength, we turn lessons into medicine, and we release what isn't ours. And for me, that is our body, in alignment with the energetics, vibrations, and frequencies of Venus.

We can work *with* the energetics, vibrations, and frequencies of Venus in so many ways, including, but not limited to: moving our bodies, entering dream temples; creating visionary art; nourishing and tending our bodies; visiting sacred sites, stones, and statues; making and receiving sound currents; connecting with nature and her rhythms, cycles, and vibrations; Sky Reading (more on this later) and astrology; ingesting plant medicine, tinctures, and herbal teas; holding ceremony and ritual.

We can attune *our* frequency, literally tune in to the 'harmonious vibration for all of creation,' also called the Venus frequency, the Ma frequency, the frequency of love. And when we come into alignment at our heart and center, we connect less to the mainstream programming of what we're being told and sold, and we become a VV – a Venusian Vessel. And well, it's here that it ALL becomes available to us. It's WONDER-FULL.

INVITATION:
CREATE A VENUS ALTAR

I invite you to keep things simple when starting to work and connect with Venus by creating a Venus altar. I love an altar because it's an intentional and devotional space to speak our power into being. While writing this book, I traveled to various locales in France, and so I created a portable Venus altar to keep by my bedside and charge up at sacred spots. I used a tin of Altoids mints for this purpose (although any small, lidded tin will work); here's what I did:

- ❖ *First, I found images online that I associate with Venus – the goddess Hathor, a wild rose, an anatomical heart, pomegranates, the Venus of Willendorf (it's important that for your altar, the talismanic items feel Venusian to you). I printed out the images, made a collage with them, and then covered the collage in clear glue before sticking it to the outside of the tin.*

- ❖ *Next, I placed a mini mirror inside the lid of the tin, on which I wrote an affirmation: I am love. I am magic. I am power. I am beauty. I am Venus. I also added a picture of myself inside the tin. You can create a port-a-altar like this to hold lil keepsakes/talismanic items by your bedside. I suggest that you too add an image of yourself as a reminder that this is in devotion to YOU, as Venus.*

Introducing the Wild Rose SHE salons

I work a LOT in the dreamtime, an art passed through my familial lineage of imaginal dream journeys. For me, it involves creating a ceremonial dream temple (where I sometimes drink heart-opening Guatemalan cacao or the Venusian plants rose, hibiscus, and blue lotus in tea form) and intentionally entering a dreamscape in which I let myself wonder *and* wander. I'm sensing and feeling what's important and what's not as I navigate the many time lines I'm weaving between.

I do this for each book I write, and during the writing of *Venus*, I got a VERY clear image of myself sat with the most interesting, powerful, funny, smart, entertaining women, some of whom had existed in history while others were archetypal female energy. We were gathered in a Parisian salon and would talk about all things Venusian – art, magic, beauty, poetry. What's NOT to love about that?

One woman who often entered my dreamtime was the real-life French writer Madeleine de Scudéry, who, in the 1640s, was the queen of the Parisian salons (gatherings held in a private home, men and women from all social classes would mingle and discuss new ideas.) Madeleine is *quite* the woman and it's through her as *salonnière* (salon hostess) that I've established my very own Secret Society of Self Source-ery: the Women of the Wild Rose. Its members are women throughout time and space who have made themselves known to me as keepers of Wild Rose medicine. And ohhh, they're golden.

The Secret Society of Self Source-ery: the Women of the Wild Rose has met (and continues to do so) for MANY tea and creativity salons in the dreamtime. And as these women all hold keys and codes for us in the here and now, I invite you to join us for six (a magic Venus number) Wild Rose SHE salons as we gather for tea and creativity. (And stargazing and dreamscaping, and magic-making.)

Why Self Source-ery? Because when we Self Source – when we slow down, listen, acknowledge, and respond to the wisdom of our sensorial, primordial nature and instinctual knowing – we're SO BLOODY POWERFUL. And when we're powerful, we REMEMBER. And when we remember, with magic and wild hope, we come in, we come down, and we SELF SOURCE.

Each of the Wild Rose SHE salons is a seductive toe dip (which, if you're anything like me, will lead to an immersive and luxurious full-body soak) into some of my favorite ways to work with Venus, her astrology, her magic, and her cycles to support you to write, re-spell, and, most importantly, live YOUR Venus story and walk (skip and/or dance) YOUR Wild Rose path.

The Venus frequency

The feminine frequency of love, the Venus frequency – the magic creative power and radiance that's been practiced and held by everyone from midwives and householders to noblewomen and queens – has been passed on. It lives within me/you/us waiting and wanting to be activated, remembered, and explored as the Wild Rose.

Women, thank the Goddess, have always found ways to gather and share. Even when it wasn't safe to (*especially* when it wasn't safe to). From back in the day when we had temples in which to cultivate our magic, power, and radiance, I can guarantee that we held rituals, rites, and ceremonies and bathed in rose- and herb-infused baths. And we can certainly recreate that today; in fact, we absolutely *should* (I share my favorite recipe for nourishing ritual tea baths on page 43.)

From the pre-Christian red tents to witches' moon circles, and through to the glorious salons of Enlightenment-era France (which often served as informal universities for women, who at the time weren't allowed to access actual universities), women have gathered and shared. Which is why I'd love you to regard me as your Wild Rose *salonnière* as I curate and create our time together.

However, it's important to be clear that I'm not teaching you anything that you don't already know. You/we ARE the mystery school. That's the point. It's IN our bodies and as we remember and trust what we know, it will become clear that we each hold different teachings and medicine that's decoded when our hearts and our souls, through our lived experiences IN our bodies, are trusted, heard, and believed.

I'll introduce you to some of the Women of the Wild Rose I've met on *my* Wild Rose path because they're amazing and I think you'll love them. But know that the women who step forward for YOU may be different because they're supporting YOU to mistress YOUR mysteries. They'll all have one thing in common, though – they'll hold a fierce (and very fabulous) feminine Venus frequency. How will you know? Oh, you'll know. You'll *feel* it and you'll want to align with it. The six Wild Rose SHE salon chapters that follow will support you to do the following:

* ❋ Build your ability, strength, and capacity to Self Source.

* ❋ Re-tell and re-spell your experience with clear intention.

* ❋ Hold and maintain your power and magic.

* ❋ Fall a little more in love with yourself, with others, with your entire life, every chance that you get by evoking and experiencing Venus – the wildest of roses – as yourself.

MY VENUS IS…

My Venus is earthy and divine.

Sublime.

Light and dark.

With an essence of sass (and snark).

My Venus has thighs that rub.

She's full.

(Of life force. Of creative sauce.)

And of course, she's soft and sensual.

And she's source.

Power.

Power that devours.

And we make love.

Often.

Between the sheets.

Of paper.

With inky red pen.

My Venus is a Wild Rose

who grows

untamed, unashamed, and she makes her own room

to bloom.

And she blooms.

And she blooms.

And she blooms.

WILD ROSE
SHE SALON

Mapping the Terrain

If you've read any of my previous books, you'll know that I'm obsessed with mapping and tracking what I call our SHE-scape – the internal and external landscape of being a woman; our lived experience through the rhythmic intelligence of cycles: of the body, the seasons, and the cosmos. And Madeleine de Scudéry, co-founder of MY Venusian woman gang, the Secret Society of Self Source-ery: the Women of the Wild Rose, was gathering with her women in Paris during the 1600s, and they were doing the EXACT same thing – mapping their felt experience.

OK, so as your *salonnière* it's only right that I tell you a little more about Madeleine. A society figure and prominent novelist who often published her work anonymously or under her brother's name, Georges, she was the first to compose a full-scale modern biography of another Wild Rose, the ancient Greek poet Sappho. Madeleine was quite the 'It girl' of her time and was accepted by some of *the* most exclusive Parisian *coteries* – groups of people who shared similar interests – before creating her own salon with like-hearts called the Société du Samedi (the Saturday Club).

In her 1654–60 novel *Clélie, or a Roman History*, Madeleine included a *Carte de Tendre* (map of love and tenderness), which charted her relationship with place and space and felt experience through the body. It's said that she created it with her Saturday salon to literally map out an answer to a question: What must one do to become a *tendre ami* (lover)?

Now THIS is the thing I want us ALL to get curious about. In fact, let it be our lifelong enquiry to each create and curate our own *Carte de Tendre*:

What must YOU do to become a *tendre ami*?

A lover. A lover of self. A lover of the entire experience of ALL OF LIFE?

We are a living map of Venus

I have passionately mapped the cyclical and rhythmic intelligence of my own felt experience for the last 17+ years and have been encouraging others to do the same, so to find Madeleine de Scudéry working in creative collaboration with other women to map emotions, creativity, and the lived experience back in the 17th freakin' century is WILD to me. And yet I also know that more than 25,000 years ago a woman's experience was being etched on the walls of a limestone rock shelter in Marquay, France; the bas-relief of a nude female now known as the Venus of Laussel holds a bison horn with notches that are said to represent both the moon and menstrual cycles.

We've *always* mapped our experiences. We've *always* told stories about them. We *need* the stories of bold and real, messy and flawed, glorious and sovereign women, Wild Roses. Not to compare but to inspire, evoke, and provoke us to trust ourselves and our own lived experiences. Venus is our invitation, through her cycles and through our bodies, to live and to tell OUR stories. To map our own emotional and felt *Carte de Tendre* and tell stories about our GREATEST adventure yet:

THIS LIFE. ME/YOU/US AS A LIVING MAP OF VENUS.

I won't lie, there have been many times throughout my life when I've very much wanted to disconnect and check out of my body – I LOVE her AND as someone who experiences Ehlers Danlos Syndrome, she's simply not always that comfortable to BE IN. (Yes, yes, I *know* that's the bloody point, but uggghhhhhhhh, it's so FUCKING FRUSTRATING.) I teach a practice called IN.YOUR.BODY.MENT – whole body support and nourishment through movement, dance, breath work, and sound practices – and the very month that I was due to launch weekly classes was the one where SHE brought me to my knees and I collapsed on the streets of Paris.

SHE said: SLOW YOUR ROLL, SWEETS – THERE'S MORE. You need to come in and come down. EVEN MORE. Be present and IN YOUR BODY. EVEN MORE. What's that? You feel like you're letting people down *again*? *Good*. Feel it IN. YOUR. BODY. EVEN MORE. What's that? You feel shame about another promise that was NOT kept? *Good*. Feel it IN. YOUR. BODY. EVEN MORE.

When I shared this experience with the women in the SHE Power Collective (my online community, which you're so welcome to join: www.lisalister.com/the-she-power-collective), many wrote to say that they too were feeling a 'collapsing' of some kind – whether it was of time lines, of beliefs, of understanding of ALL. THE. BLOODY. THINGS. And this is how it is for us Wild Roses; we'll experience these moves and shakes in different ways AND there will *always* be similarities.

Personally, I was *really* pissed off because I *had* spent the previous few years really SLOWING DOWN, allowing more of *me* to 'become' in the knowledge that we're all 'perpetually becoming.' I even wrote a book about it, called *Self Source-ery*. And yet there I was in that time of chaos – the space I refer to as the 'mother of creation' – being called to slow down EVEN MORE. To witness that the *real* flex is to see and feel into rest *as* action. Rest *as* expansion. Rest *as* renewal and possibility. I DID NOT/STILL DO NOT LIKE IT. And yet… I was going to write 'I had no choice' but we *always* have choice. And so I CHOSE to surrender, and that, ultimately, was the path back to my power.

The slowdown

My nervous system was calling me to Self Source EVEN MORE – past what felt 'socially acceptable.' To not simply claim 'I'm better' but to really rest enough for it to nourish me, cell-deep. But I had so much to DO. So many plans, a life to live. And let's be real, bills to pay. Yet I couldn't do *any* of those things without being Self Source-ed.

Only I thought I *had* Self Source-ed. I thought I *had* slowed down. I thought I *was* listening to my body. But SHE said, through my body: slow down EVEN MORE. Tend to, nourish, and Self Source EVEN MORE. Listen EVEN MORE. And it was/is so frustrating because I knew that I'd been hanging on tightly to anxiety. I had a story, a really good one, that told me: *This is how we get things done*, and I realized, in the slowdown, that I was actually scared that *without* anxiety, I'd do nothing. If I tended to my nervous system to a point of *true* rest and relaxation, well… I'd DO NOTHING.

It's as if I *never* wanted to let it be easy. I'd *always* do the thing for which I had a deadline rather than the thing that brought me total joy and pleasure. (And that's how so many of us have been taught to survive in Western society. The power of the guilt that we feel when we *choose* joy and pleasure over the thing we've been 'paid' to do is often so heavy that it no longer feels joyful or pleasurable to actually do it.)

So, I DID rest. And when I'm in a state of change (which as a Wild Rose, you WILL start to recognize as a phase of power) I like to return to what's familiar. It helps me anchor into what I KNOW, and in this particular scenario that looked like eating a metric shit ton of collagen-infused bone broth, taking a lot of healing herb-infused baths, and reading (and rereading) the poems written by a 14th-century North Indian mystic called Lalla.

I LOVE Lalla. She was a lioness, a truth teller, a courageous woman who sang songs of naked awareness in medieval Kashmir. (This woman was BADASS and also clearly a Wild Rose.) My fave version of her work has been translated by Coleman Barks in the book *Naked Song* and I particularly love the following lines, which are tattooed on my heart:

> *I went everywhere, with longing in my eyes.*
> *Until here, in my own house, I felt truth filling my sight.*

It was here that SLOW became my practice. I'd often written about 'slow living'; about how I really like the IDEA of it and how, at some points in my life I actually believed I *was* slow living. Except I absolutely wasn't. So, I started to consider what I *thought* I meant by 'slow living,' and it began with being more INTENTIONAL about how I spend my time. Focusing on quality over quantity. Finding joy and pleasure in the simple things.

So far, so thoroughly self-help-y, right?! Like something someone who has the time to bake and sew, pack the kids' lunch boxes, batch cook at the weekend, and y'know, DO ALL THE THINGS would say. Except, I *really* DID want to live my life that way (and not be one of *those* hipster wankers in the process, although I'm not entirely sure that's actually possible! *Wink*.)

So, then I asked, which word encompasses all of that? I really like *devotional*, but I believe that pretty much everything about the way I live my life is devotional – it's how I choose to move. But what does devotional and intentional slowdown look and *feel* like? *Savoring* – the slow and pleasurable appreciation of positive experiences. Yep, another lesson learned from the French – savoring became my THING.

Practicing the art of savoring

When I savor life, I'm present, in the moment, to fully experience ALL of life. I started drinking coffee from my Paris teacup because it was fancy, and it made me feel special at a time when I wasn't feeling particularly special. I witnessed the ways in which I'd pushed some of my bigger dreams aside, dreams that my soul yearned and longed for, because I literally had no energy.

So, I made a list of the things that depleted that energy supply, and I got intentional about letting go and releasing *everything* on that list. It included people – yep, I REALLY went there – situations, certain work things that I did because I'm a control freak and hadn't been able to let go of. And also, the amount of fucking time I'd given to worrying/fretting about things that have never ACTUALLY happened. I. WAS. SO. OVER. IT. Prioritizing my well-being and taking *actual* care of myself was/is FIERCE Self Source-ery. It's LOVE IN ACTION.

So, now I savor. I LIKE savoring. I think my internalized bias against slow said it was boring – and that if *I* was slow, I was lazy. That's OLD PARADIGM shit right there, isn't it?! So, I'm still getting comfy with 'slow,' but in the meantime, 'to savor life' feels way 'sexier' to my Scorpio nature. (Yep, leave it to a Scorpio to 'sex up' the situ. ANY situ.)

To savor feels intentional – it's on purpose and it makes the experience of life-living, well… a little bit more bloody delicious. AND I DO still give a fuck, but now, more than ever, I'm REALLY specific about to who and where I *give* those fucks because they are DEFINITELY much sparser than they have been in the last few years. Ha!

NOTE: My nanna would always say 'this too shall pass,' but when you're IN IT – and for many of us, 'it' can look like so many different things: health issues, a trauma, depression, burnout, wherever and whenever it might feel bloody dark – it's really hard to believe that you'll have enough energy/interest/passion/enthusiasm to DO all the things EVER again.

For me, in that particular health situ, it meant I got curious, because really that's all there ever is to DO when you're in it. My workload, the things I'd said 'yes' to BP (Before Paris), were already starting to lean toward potential overwhelm, so when I tuned in, my body was saying:

Refine MORE.

Define MORE.

Align MORE.

It's a feminine art and superpower to KNOW that the chaos and not-knowing of these wild and shifting times is, like the goddess Kali Ma, pure creative essence. Destructive, yes… AND regenerative and creative and supporting new possibilities and opportunities for us to evolve and grow.

Trusting our knowing

The 'invitation' (that's in inverted commas because it's ALWAYS an invitation, and yet you KNOW it's actually a soul command) is to TRUST that in these experiences of destruction AND creative regeneration, your heart, your deepest ALL-SEEING KNOWING, has something WAY juicier planned. What if you dared to trust THAT?

Now, it can definitely be hard to trust *that* when it feels like things are coming to a head and life is potentially falling apart. But, and bear with me on this one, what if we think of it as an update on our phone – inconvenient and annoying, but ultimately supporting a smoother, less glitchy experience in the future. In my case, SHE had me slow all the way down so that I could REMEMBER what it is that I KNOW.

She was right: I DID know that what I *was* doing was NOT it, and yet… it was VERY alluring. Because of my background, I've always needed to figure out how to survive. And the idea of creating my own reality, of daring and then letting myself be nourished by what I love, in service to love, in order to really bloody thrive? Well, that's still *very* new to me. And yet my heart and my soul KNOWS this as truth.

Yes, she had to take me out at the knees (but she DID do it in Paris, and she DID send the hot pompiers) so that I could recalibrate and realign with that question:

What must one do to become a *tendre ami* (lover)?

My response? Right now (knowing that it can, and inevitably will, change):

* I must open my heart as wide as it'll go and move, as the poet and Wild Rose Mary Oliver suggests, 'with the rhythms that feel true to my own essence.'

* I must tend to and love on my body as both divinity AND human form.

* I must recalibrate and realign with MY heart, with what MATTERS.

* I must honor my desires and truly savor them – art, poetry, words, travel, dance, magic, and wonder – as *my* Wild Rose path.

It makes space for *more* of my magic, power, and wisdom to become available – *that's* how it works. I magnetize more of what it is I tend to and I savor it, I *truly* savor it with ALL of my senses. It fills me up and it satiates, sources, and supports me to TRULY thrive. To be in the poetics of being FULLY ALIVE. As a living map of Venus.

I wish this for you too, with ALL MY BIG, BEAT-Y WILD ROSE HEART.

Cleopatra, Venus, and bathing rituals

To me, there's no better way to practice savoring than to bathe, and there's no one more fitting to teach us about bathing than Wild Rose Cleopatra, Pharaoh of Egypt and empress of MY heart. There are so many reasons why I love her but let me list a few. Referred to as a 'scheming siren' by some – of course she was – she was also nicknamed 'Venus' by many others.

Cleopatra was super smart; she spoke more than 20 languages, and you'd better believe she used her beauty, charm, *and* smarts to negotiate with other leaders. She identified with many deities, all of whom held the Venus frequency, but her favorite was Isis, and she'd often dress as the goddess, fully taking on her essence and her power.

NOTE: THIS is a Venus superpower – recognizing ourselves *as* Venus, *as* deity, so that we can realize and recognize the source power that resides within us, our wants and desires as source, as Goddess. So that we become our own greatest lover.

Cleopatra *knew* the power of the senses. Not only would she wear the very best perfumes on her body, but it's also said that when meeting her lover, Marc Antony, she'd soak the sails of her ships with fragrant oils so that her presence in scent form would arrive on the shore before she did. Legend also says that a herd of 700 lactating donkeys provided the milk for her daily rose-petal, milk, and herb baths. I MEAN!

Now, I very much fancy myself as a modern-day Cleopatra, always have, not least because I too often bathe in an infusion of milk and roses. Thankfully, for my preferred blend, NO donkeys are required – hurrah! In fact, it was passed down from my nanna, who bathed me in it when I was a baby to relieve my eczema. And today, any time I get a flare-up, or simply need the remembrance of Ma magic and love (or feel the need to embody Cleo, which is often), I return to it.

I'm aware that I have a *lot* of water in my natal/birth astrology chart but bathing and soaking, especially in an herbal infusion, is one of my favorite rituals of devotion, intention, savor, and support. And I'm not alone. The practice, often called 'tea bathing' because essentially, the bathtub becomes a big ol' teacup of herbs infused in hot water, was used by the ancient Babylonians, Egyptians, Greeks, Romans, and Japanese.

INVITATION:
RUN A ROSE AND MILK TEA BATH

For tens of thousands of years, tea bathing has been used as a hygiene ritual, as a show of deep respect for divinity, as a spiritual practice, and as a tool for self-healing.

What you'll need

Two small drawstring muslin bags (I make my own, but you can buy them and they're reusable) each filled with a handful of the following ingredients:

- *Dried rose buds and petals – useful as an anti-inflammatory, these evoke feelings of love and luxe.*

- *Dried calendula flowers – anti-inflammatory, antimicrobial, antibacterial, soothing, and analgesic, this plant promotes rapid healing.*

- *Dried lavender flowers – these will invigorate your overall mood, combat stress, and relieve muscle tension.*

- *Dried chamomile flowers – these are antibacterial and help to reduce redness and to minimize scars and marks.*

What to do

1. To one of the 'teabags' add a handful of oats and then place that teabag in a running bath and let it steep for eight to 10 minutes. Place the other teabag in a cup and add hot water: Yep, we're pairing a drinking tea with your tea bath – love for both the inside and outside. I also add two cups of raw milk to the bath because it exfoliates, softens, and smooths the skin by removing dead skin cells. But if you're vegan or would simply prefer not to use milk, you can replace it with a hefty handful of coconut milk powder.

2. Next, set a clear intention for the bath. Mine is often to soften, to receive love, and to heal. Get in the bath and bring your cup of tea infusion with you. With each sip of the tea, allow yourself to soften, to be open to receive love and to heal (or whatever your intention is for the bath.) When you're complete, let the bathwater drain fully, taking with it anything that needs to be released, before getting out of the bath.

An extra: After your bath, stand in front of a mirror and whisper words of love to each of your body parts as you dry them – the body wants nothing more than for us to show her love and attention!

Smell the roses!

My nanna always smelled of roses and she made her own rose water, which is still my favorite thing to create and smell too. I make it from my Ma lineage rose – it was in my nanna's garden, then in my mumma's garden, and now it's in mine. And rose water is something we can make in dedication and devotion to Venus. It smells delicious and you can use it for so many things. I add it to my morning coffee; I put some in my ceremonial cacao for a heart-opening drink; I put it in a spritz bottle and use it as a morning face mist (I started this when my skin would get super inflamed and now I do it just because it smells and feels lush.)

And, like Marie Antoinette, the queen of France during the French Revolution of the late 18th century, I also use it as a pillow spray. Marie Antoinette would have someone spray her bedroom and pillows with rose and jasmine before she woke in the morning – how decadent is THAT? If, unlike Marie Antoinette, you *don't* live with servants or willing partners, then be your own queen and spray your own pillows. It's said that she, like Cleopatra, would also take daily baths in rose infusions. It's clearly a QUEEN THING.

NOTE: Marie Antoinette was a Wild Rose, too. Now, she certainly wasn't perfect – who is?! – but she most definitely was misunderstood and defamed. For example, she did NOT say 'let them eat cake.' That phrase was one that French citizens had been attributing to the foreign queens of French kings for DECADES before her reign. According to Caroline Weber in her book *Queen of Fashion: What Marie Antoinette Wore to the Revolution*, it's because they had a 'displaced frustration with the crown.'

Yes, Marie Antoinette *did* love the finer things in life; in true Venusian style, she thoroughly celebrated art, beauty, and poetry, and she refused to drink anything but hot chocolate – a woman after my own heart. And like me, she had a Venus in Scorpio placement. So, you'd better believe she didn't apologize for being queen; in fact, it's said that she rarely, if ever, apologized for anything.

Controversially, I love Marie Antoinette. As with so many of the women who have been labelled 'notorious' and blamed and shamed throughout the ages, I believe that the 'good girl programming' which so many of us are in the process of unpicking could learn a lot from her audacious and unapologetic nature.

What are YOU tired of apologizing for?

Where, if anywhere, are you spending time trying to be 'liked,' to the detriment of your art, your power, and your magic?

INVITATION:
MAKE YOUR OWN ROSE WATER

Of course, you can buy rose water, but if you, like my nanna and me, want to make your own, let me share how I do it.

NOTE: *While I was in Northern France charting my rose lines, I made a special batch of French 'wild rose' water. Yep, wild roses grow in hedgerows there, and I collected the petals when they bloomed in early June. You've got to be quick, because a wild rose usually only flowers for about two weeks. You can make rose water from any of your favorite rose sources, although I do recommend picking the petals in the morning to get the best harvest. You can also collect the rosehips any time after the first hard frost of the season to make teas, medicine, and syrup.*

What you'll need

A heatproof bowl; a large saucepan with a lid; five cups of water; one cup of dried rose petals or two cups of fresh rose petals; ice cubes.

What to do

1. *Place the heatproof bowl in the center of the saucepan. Add the water and the rose petals to the pan around the bowl (making sure nothing gets inside the bowl). Place the lid on the pan upside down, and then bring the water to a boil.*

2. *Reduce the heat to a simmer and then add a few ice cubes to the top of the pan lid. As the ice melts, pour off the water and add more ice. Continue this process until the color fades from the rose petals and a quantity of clean, clear rose water has collected inside the bowl.*

3. *Allow everything to cool before bottling and using.*

Rose water's magical properties are perfect for balancing an open heart with having strong boundaries; and it can assist you in finding a healthy balance between being in action and being relaxed. For those of us who try to control and overthink EVERYTHING (Hi, that's me), rose water offers relaxation; and it can be super supportive to spritz yourself and/or the room you're in if you're someone who is constantly busy or who can't slow down as a part of a trauma response. Sigh.

Rose, as medicine and healer, like Venus, is the great harmonizer, and it can be used to help us come into alignment with our big, beat-y hearts. It supports us to become the *tendre ami*, the lover, and to choose the Venus frequency, the frequency of love.

EVERY. SINGLE. TIME.

Magdalene Medicine – love in action

What I'm *slowly* starting to realize and recognize is that all this – the mapping and tracking of our rhythmic intelligence, love in ALL its forms, the poetics of aliveness, the tending, nourishing, satiating, and celebrating of our body as both divine AND human – is Magdalene Medicine. ALL. OF. IT.

I talk about Mary Magdalene in all my books. Everything I do, write, draw, and share is infused with HER. So, of course it's ALL HER medicine. HER siren call. To me/you/us as her 21st-century PR women to re-write the story. HER story. Our story. To BE love in action THROUGH our bodies.

Despite what we've been told, as shared by the glorious Meggan Watterson in her book *Mary Magdalene Revealed* (read it, it's GORGEOUS), we were never meant to transcend the body – the body is NOT sinful, we ARE worthy, and we need NOTHING outside of ourselves. It's all IN OUR BODY. And because it's never an either/or situation but a 'this and that' one, we're divine as fuck. We're so bloody messy and well, human, AND we're divine.

The ask is for us to REMEMBER. I think this is super clear to read in the Magdalene gospel (the gospel that they tried to keep from us because it was considered 'dangerous' and would contradict *everything* they've wanted us to believe: that women aren't powerful, that we need someone outside ourselves to save us, that the body is sinful, and… well, you get the idea.)

And I'm finding it through my own fascinating encounters with many of the Women of the Wild Rose; for example, did you know that many believed Joan of Arc was Magdalene reincarnated? In fact, ALL the women I'm ever called to share – Cassandra, Cleopatra, Madonna, Miley Cyrus – carry the

Magdalene Medicine. We ALL carry the Magdalene thread. THAT is why we're here, TOGETHER, in the Secret Society of Self Source-ery. Gathered as Women of the Wild Rose. Because WE. ARE. SO. BLOODY. POWERFUL.

We carry the thread of *every* Magdalene – remembering that she's a woman, *and* she's a frequency, *and* she's an archetype, *and* she's a mystery school, *and* she's a mythos, *and* she's a transmission. Every woman, real or archetypal, who has been maligned, not believed, objectified, silenced, censored, blamed and shamed, 'fallen' and been 'redeemed' (can you feel the burn?!) – it's ALL Magdalene Medicine.

We experience this in our body, we watch others experience it, and we REALLY FEEL THE BLOODY BURN. So that the stories, all that we're told and sold, all the shame and blame we've carried as our own, can burn away and we remember who the fuck we are.

It's what Mary Magdalene wants for us all.

That we remember who SHE was (love and power and magic and Venus. Pure mother-loving divine love and power and magic and Venus.)

So that we remember and trust who WE are. (Love and power and magic and Venus. Pure mother-loving divine love and power and magic and Venus.)

To remember and KNOW that we are not sinful, we are divine.

We are love. PURE love.

And as we remember, we become aligned.

IN our body, with our heart and soul. Refined, defined, AND aligned with our true and real nature so that the inevitable miracles and magic rebirth. Over and over.

SHE speaks ancient-future, and she wants you/us to remember that you/we do too. (Because YOU are SHE and SHE is YOU.) So, it's ALL a remembering. AND it's already happened. AND it's yet to come. SHE reminds us that deeper doesn't always mean dark, as in not visible, because we *can* see in the dark, remember? THIS is the mistress-ry. Discovered only by being IN the body AND IN the mystery. AT THE SAME TIME. And remembering that you/we are the mistresses of the mystery.

Rise rooted

Like the Wild Rose, you're rooted. Soft. And strong. You're living in your feelings space, in the sensory information that speaks through you to guide your next moves. In alignment with your heart and all that it desires. Moving moment to moment – not too far into the future and not too far back into the fears, worries, and grief of the past – and totally present in the here and now.

It's *not* a relationship with your 'higher self' because personally, I don't believe there's any part of us that's 'better' or 'higher.' But there is *so* much more capacity for aliveness in the body when we're in alignment with ALL OF OUR PARTS. When we're whole. When we follow the cues and clues of our most aligned and whole self (she's SO FREAKING WISE), our next move is always creating *with* Venus.

It's a total trust in life being harmonized so that we're an embodied and sourced force that attracts and receives the relationships, the collaborative projects, the partners, the money that are/is a vibrational match (knowing that this will be different for each of us). So that we can really love life and it can love us right back.

It's how we stay rooted in our body AND how we're able to dream and create. It's how we're both visionary AND practical. These Times? They've been prophesied as a period of change and transition, and we can look to all the places in our own lives where we too have experienced change and transition. Where the cycles of nature, including those of Venus herself, have built-in phases that we can CHOOSE to enter, and which provide a supportive container to Self Source.

So that we can trust ourselves to navigate the terrain of these wild and shifting times as a whole human, a sourced force – emotionally, physically, mentally, and spiritually – who can hold and contain her magic, power, and expansion, maintain balance and harmony, and dream an entire new future/ possibility/experience into being.

Yes, you've experienced tough and dark times, AND you choose to live and embody love.

Yes, challenges will STILL occur, and they will help you to keep aligning, defining, and refining with what REALLY matters.

Yes, you WILL become more magnetic – that's how this works. So, direct your compass toward all that is an energetic match for your power, magic, and medicine in the knowing that you WILL have to filter out and keep filtering out outdated beliefs and the opinions of others, so that you remain and sustain *your* Venus vibration.

When you're heart-centered and Venus-led, you're a sourced force who can dream, create, and initiate YOUR reality.

Follow your Wild Rose petaled path

Smell the roses

As my nanna always said, stop and smell the roses. Actual and/or metaphorical ones. Slow down – ALL. THE. WAY. DOWN – and savor. Let yourself become satiated and sourced by all of life.

Become a tendre ami (lover)

What MUST you do to become a lover of the entire experience of life? Make this a lifelong enquiry. Make a devotional list and have the very best fun and adventures discovering YOUR Venus love language.

Align, refine, define

Let your rhythmic intelligence keep meeting at your heart, in the frequency of love and all things Venus, to map and continually re-map the terrain. To fully live in the poetics of FULL aliveness.

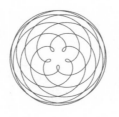

Be in the poetics of
aliveness as a living
map of Venus.

WILD ROSE
SHE SALON

Venus Astrology

'Let's lose the watch and live by the pulse alone.'
NATALIE CLIFFORD BARNEY, AMERICAN WRITER

Many of us know our 'big three' astrological signs – our sun, moon, and rising signs, right? But for me personally, really getting to know my astrological Venus placement (more on this coming up) and the way it impacts my relationships with myself and with others – as well as with money and pleasure – has been a total game-changer in HOW I navigate my life.

Venus's astrological symbol is a mirror, and she wants us to be self-reflective. When I talk about Venus as a feminine frequency, for me it starts here: coming into connection with Venus in our natal (or birth) chart. But before we do this together, I can't wait to introduce you to another member of the Secret Society of Self Source-ery: the poet, author, and lover of life Natalie Clifford Barney (1876–1972), who, it's said, in true Wild Rose style, 'never belonged to anyone but herself.'

Born in the USA, Natalie later relocated to Paris, where, like Madeleine de Scudéry before her, she founded a women's society, l'Académie des Femmes (Women's Academy), in 1927. According to the blog www.messynessychic.com, for Natalie, 'life overflowed with color, creativity, and passion in Paris's Left Bank during one of the city's most romantic periods.' Sigh.

One of the reasons I love Natalie so much is because, as Suzannah Rodriguez explains in her biography *Wild Heart, A Life: Natalie Clifford Barney's Journey from Victorian America to the Literary Salons of Paris* (read it, you will NOT regret it), she was a 'devotee of astrology and numerology who formed a club of friends called "The Scorpions" after their shared astrological symbol.'

And in true witch style, the club would meet on October 31 each year and Natalie would wear a long velvet gown 'emblazoned with astrological signs.' (I don't know about you, but I now very much believe that we all NEED a long velvet gown covered in astrological signs. I'm going to go hot pink velvet with metallic copper symbology. You?)

Natalie had a temple in her garden where – you've guessed it – wild roses would grow among the lilacs and everyone from Gertrude Stein to Colette and Truman Capote visited. She was a lesbian who took a lot of lovers (high fives to that!) and wore her hair long and wild at a time when such things were considered scandalous. All this is why I lovingly refer to her as the 'notorious NCB,' and she and I bond the most over our shared Venus in Scorpio placement – intense, magnetic, passionate, and powerful.

Venus in your natal chart

Venus in your natal or birth chart is YOUR magnetic frequency. It can show you all that you need to know about your relationships: with yourself, with others, and with lovers; with beauty and art, fashion and style; with your self-worth and your values and beliefs. And it will shine a light on how you interact with money, with pleasure, with all that brings you joy. Natal

Venus is the key to HOW you live and experience your life in its fullest expression.

Venus rules the astrological signs of Taurus and Libra and while both are associated with luxe, money, aesthetics, and style, they each hold different qualities of Venus. For example, Taurus holds the Venus traits of our relationship with ourselves – the senses, sensuality, physical needs, self-worth, trust, values (both spiritual and material); while Libra holds the Venus traits of our relationships with others – our friends, colleagues, and lovers – and our relationship with resources, justice, harmony, beauty, and peace.

Knowing where Venus is for you, in your natal chart, can offer up the insight YOU need to explore all the things that Venus is best known for: love, relationships, beauty, creativity, style, and money. It can also help you to get better acquainted with what it is you're most attracted to and why (as well as what you're *currently* attracting and why. It's magnetism. And Venus is ALL ABOUT IT!), as well as your gifts and resources (and how to utilize them in a way that creates the most pleasure and joy. Yep, Venus wants us to stop making it so bloody hard for ourselves and actively encourages us to let it be easy.) And most importantly, how to make life-living a delicious and creative and harmonious art form.

NOTE: I'm what's known in the Gypsy/Traveller tradition as a 'Sky Reader.' Like my mumma before me and my nanna before her, I'm not overly concerned with the angles and degrees of astrology. Instead, I 'feel' the planets and constellations in my body and know their correspondences with the seasons. As the ancient temple priestesses of Hathor did in Egypt's Dendera temple, I literally read the sky through felt experience. This is what our ancestors did for millennia, and temples were created for this specific purpose.

Today, we can study all the branches of astrology – I have and still do – yet the way I do it is a bit less formal and a LOT more intuition- and instinct-led. My mumma taught me how to find the constellations in the sky, how to know what the moon was doing at any given moment, and to witness Venus as both evening and morning star (and to feel the difference of both in my body), which is where my love for all things Venus began.

I share this because, personally, I find the traditional Western astrological tradition of 'You're a Scorpio, so…' a little constrictive (although having said that, I *am* a Scorpio, and I am all the things that Western astrology associates with a Scorpio, so I WILL also contradict myself!) But in *this* SHE salon, I want to let Western astrology be our starting point, while recognizing that it has its limitations. And then, if you're called, we can always dive further together into Sky Reading in real time. Deal?

Find and interpret your Venus placement

Your natal/birth chart is a snapshot of what the sky looked like – the positions of the planets – at the exact moment you were born. If you already know how to read your birth chart and find your Venus placement, awesome. But if you don't, begin by searching online for a natal/birth chart generator/ calculator or download an astrology app and put in the details that the system asks for – it'll usually be the time, date, and place of your birth.

This will generate your natal birth chart. Good news is that most online generators and phone apps offer both a visual map and a written summary that will tell you exactly which astrological sign and house each planet is in (*see below*). In our work together, though, we're only looking at Venus.

To find YOUR Venus placement – the astrological sign and house that Venus was in the moment you entered Earth side – start by looking for the symbol that resembles a handheld mirror on your natal chart; it will be, at most, two astrological signs behind or ahead of your sun sign.

The astrological signs and houses

A natal/birth chart is split into 12 sections, with each section representing a different way for the planets to express themselves (the astrological signs) *and* a particular aspect/ theme of life (the astrological houses). As the planets shift and change, they occupy both an astrological sign and a house, creating a unique pattern for every one of us. Your first house is your rising sign, and that's calculated using your time, date, and place of birth. From there, you follow the houses anticlockwise around the zodiac wheel, from 1 to 12.

If you're new to astrology, here's a simple visual guide to the astrological symbols, signs, houses, and elements.

Symbol	Sign	House	Element
♈	Aries	1st House of Self	Fire
♉	Taurus	2nd House of Value and Possessions	Earth
♊	Gemini	3rd House of Communication	Air
♋	Cancer	4th House of Family and Home	Water

Symbol	Sign	House	Element
♌	Leo	5th House of Pleasure	Fire
♍	Virgo	6th House of Health	Earth
♎	Libra	7th House of Partnerships	Air
♏	Scorpio	8th House of Transformation	Water
♐	Sagittarius	9th House of Purpose	Fire
♑	Capricorn	10th House of Social Status	Earth
♒	Aquarius	11th House of Friendships	Air
♓	Pisces	12th House of Subconscious	Water

As Venus moves around the zodiac wheel, she visits every astrological sign and with her occupation of each one, she'll cast her influence on the house in which she was at the time of your birth - this is called her placement.

To interpret YOUR Venus placement, use this formula: The planet (Venus) is expressed through the astrological sign (Gemini) in the aspect/theme of the 4th house - family and home. So, if I were interpreting the Venus placement of Gemini in the 4th house for someone, the formula would be: Venus (planet of love, self-worth, values) is expressing herself through the astrological sign of Gemini (communication) in the 4th house, which is family and home, nurturing and sensitivity.

From that, I'd see that it's important for the person to be able to feel comfortable enough to openly say how they feel in any moment, especially with family and those they live with.

So, when looking up your own Venus placement, be sure to read both your Venus sign *and* your Venus house and then let what you discover help create your own Venus story.

Venus in the astrological signs and houses

What I share about Venus as she presents in each astrological sign and house is not intended to be definitive. No. Where. Near. You may identify with *some* of it, and you may totally disagree with other parts. I try not to see any of our astrological placements as diagnostic – we're the sum of *all* our parts and your Venus placement will be affected by the other planetary placements in your chart.

My suggestion? Don't overcomplicate things. Astrology can be technical and specific and sometimes confusing, and I like to keep it as simple as possible, because like my mumma, I care WAY more about how it *feels*.

Venus in a Fire sign: Aries, Leo, Sagittarius

You're hot, passionate, and exciting and you love hard and fast. You love to live life at a rapid pace and seek the thrills (and edges and risks). You're always ready for, and initiating, new adventures.

Venus in an Earth sign: Taurus, Virgo, Capricorn

You find the most joy in the smallest pleasures – a cup of delicious coffee, slow and sensual touch, smelling the roses. You have an eye for detail and a love of luxury and high-quality items, including fabrics, bed sheets, ALL THE PRETTY THINGS. You are ALL about the sensual experience – touch, hold, smell, and feel (and the literal pleasure of sex).

Venus in an Air sign: Gemini, Libra, Aquarius

You connect with others and are aroused by whispered words of love and intellectual conversation. You love to experience ALL the possibilities through play and having fun. You're sociable and want to share all that you love with those you love.

Venus in a Water sign: Cancer, Scorpio, Pisces

You prefer your connections to be deep and heart-centered, with fewer words and more feels. Your sensitive and empathic nature means that you feel and experience the emotions of life fully. You're very receptive and expressive, and while it may take you a little longer to fall in love, when you do, it's deep and you mean it.

Venus ♀ in Aries ♈ or the 1st House of Self

Ahhh, I already know that you know about love at first sight because this placement is ALL about falling in love first and falling in love fast. You love to love, and you *always* want that love to be a forever love. Until the next time you fall in love, that is. And then the next time.

Of course, this *fast love* applies to other humans, as well as to places, things, ideas, a song, a movie, a concept. You're an unapologetically passionate human (and there's NOTHING wrong with that) and that fire burns fast and bright. So, you attract like-hearts and prefer to be in relationships – both love and work – with those who can 'keep up' and meet you there.

You make bold moves in life – whether it's the clothes you wear, the career you pursue, the love affairs you experience – you take risks, you aren't afraid to make mistakes, and you're all the way in. If something *isn't* for you (and you know this based on whether it makes you feel alive and fills you with excitement), then you dismiss it and move on to the next thing, pronto.

You make money best by igniting both your own passion and the passion in others; being self-employed; taking risks; and working independently. You may often be 'too hot to handle,' but your job is to make sure that the passionate fire doesn't burn out (and in the process, burn you out.) Work with your passion spark and you can ignite a creative fire that will provide enough energy and momentum to turn all your ideas into your actual reality.

Venus ♀ in Taurus ♉ or the 2nd House of Values and Possessions

Taurus is one of Venus's two astrological home signs, so you'd better believe that her Venusian frequencies are amped up in *this* placement. You have a glorious appetite for the luxe-y things in life – good food, scents, places and spaces, lovely fabrics, gorgeous experiences – and you feel them all THROUGH your senses.

Yep, your sensorial nature is both a gift and an art form because with this placement you use ALL your senses to fully taste and savor the entire experience of life, including pleasure. You know that feeling safe, having stability, and being IN the body is how you're most receptive to love.

So, it may take you a while to figure out what and/or who it is you DO like and value – you're a slow burn – but when you *do*, you sign up and you stay loyal. Whether it's to a person, to a brand, or a standard of living. It's why you make money best by investing in people and property, where your wealth will accumulate over time. When you're led by your senses, you take it slow, you savor each moment, and you fully experience every sensual drop of life so that more pleasure can be present, for longer, in your body. Yummm.

Venus ♀ in Gemini ♓ or the 3rd House of Communication

Ohhhh, now this placement is one of flirty banter – flanter. Whispered words, a strong text game, songs sung, poems written, books shared, intimate and stimulating conversation: These are like the most delicious foreplay to you. You're a social butterfly and prefer to make love with your mind and through the art of conversation and words (and sometimes even a heated debate) before you even entertain the idea of physical touch.

Most of your money is spent on travel, socializing, and communicating, so you'll probably have the most up-to-date phone and laptop combo and your next trip away already booked. And if you can turn this into your work and business? EVEN BETTER. Intelligence, forever learning, and a never-satiated curiosity are a complete turn-on for you.

And if the plan is for you to stick around – and let's be honest, you *are* easily bored, and you *do* tend to change your mind – it's actually a requirement. (That goes for romantic encounters, life experiences, *and* work-based activities: If your mind isn't stimulated, no matter how visually appealing the 'offer' may be, it'll be a 'no.' Love you for that.)

Venus ♀ in Cancer ♋ or the 4th House of Family and Home

You love to love, and to be loved by someone with a Venus in Cancer placement – one of *the* most nurturing placements – is to be REALLY BLOODY LOVED. Once your heart is open, you go all in. However, that rarely happens instantly – in fact, you may tend to put up a tough, self-protective shell to people and experiences until you feel comfy, safe, and 'at home' in their presence.

This is totally understandable: You have a tender underbelly and are more sensitive than most to heartbreak and rejection. Whether it's a person, a passion, a place and space, or an experience, you're ALL ABOUT IT, and while you might consider holding back in life and love because of the fear of potential heartbreak, you also know that when you DO dare to take a chance on love, in all its forms, the rewards are worth it.

You're led by your emotions, you love to make memories, and you're super sentimental. You're also majorly skilled at creating a sense of 'home' in any situation – whether that's putting a lover's mind at ease, arranging the furniture in a way that makes it welcoming to others, investing in property, working specifically with women, whispering words of encouragement to a friend in need, or simply baking a cake… because let's be honest, we ALL love cake!

Venus ♀ in Leo ♌ or the 5th House of Pleasure

You're a playful, passionate, and pleasure-seeking provocateur who loves to be adored, and you're often the center of attention. Rarely one to shy away from the limelight, you love public shows of affection, and you love to be praised for a job well done. And let's be clear, you'd take major offense if someone suggested keeping any type of celebration involving you – a birthday, a launch, an anniversary – 'low key.'

You're a fiery Creatrix and are forever creating your own scenes and narratives in life because you have a unique and magical view and perspective of the world. It's NO surprise that Dita Von Teese, the Queen of Burlesque, has a Venus in Leo placement and this is how you can make the most money – by living your best bold, beautiful, and creative life.

Charismatic, charming, and super seductive, you take ALL that you're passionate about in life VERY seriously. Ambivalence and mediocrity are NOT in your vocabulary and whether it's your wardrobe, your art, your work, or your approach to love, one thing's for sure, it'll NEVER be boring.

Venus ♀ in Virgo ♍ or the 6th House of Health

If you have this placement, some *might* say that you're 'fussy.' Not me, though: I'd call you discerning, and detail-orientated. *Wink*. In fact, I think it's bloody brilliant that you'd rather go without than spend your precious time, money, and/or energy on a person/place/situation that doesn't meet, and more importantly, respect, you for who you are and what you're about. In fact, you'll rarely if ever go back to a person, place, or situation if you're not respected – and high fives to you for THAT.

But when you DO fall in love with a person, place, project – and you'll usually know that based on how it feels in your body, because you're very body aware – you're generous, you show up to it fully, and you're present to the entire experience.

While public shows of affection are not necessarily your 'thing,' you really respond to simple gestures and details – the thought given to a gift, a bowl of soup when you're sick, or the book recommendation based on an earlier conversation. And it's how you show your love and affection, too: through acts of love and service.

Venus ♀ in Libra ♎ or the 7th House of Partnerships

Libra is one of the two signs of the zodiac that Venus rules and so you'd better believe that she shines big and bright in this placement. You're a total charmer who loves to love, and your superpower is your ability to harmonize any situation. Dealing with conflict, however, is most definitely not a strength.

Now, no one's saying you need to be argumentative, but you *are* allowed to disagree; in fact, you can create balance in all your relationships - familial, work, financial, romantic - by using your diplomacy and your need for fairness to practice respectfully challenging ideas and concepts. Cooperation is good but compromising to the detriment of your own experience is not.

From hosting parties and curating a beautiful social media feed to the products you use when taking a bath, pleasure and beauty are more than simply a lifestyle choice for you - you live for them. (And you love it even more when others, especially those you're in relationship with, notice them too.) This is THE most perfect way for you to make money - through socializing, relating to others, and communication.

Venus ♀ in Scorpio ♏ or the 8th House of Transformation

There's *nothing* casual about you, is there? You're all or nothing when it comes to being in relationship with others. Your penetrating power precedes you and it can feel pretty intense – UNDERSTATEMENT – some might even say intimidating, to be in your presence. And… well, turns out that's *just* the way you like it. Those with a Venus in Scorpio placement are renowned for their power gaze – it's ALL in the eyes.

You're motivated by wanting and needing a deep intimacy and transformational experience with all things Venusian – if there isn't an opportunity for real and deep soul growth, chances are it will be of no interest to you. And that matters because that's the area where it's most beneficial for you to make money: transformation.

You're mysterious and secretive because let's be clear, trust doesn't come easily to you. But when there *is* trust (and that may or may not come after much super sleuthing and scoping out *everything* there is to know about the person/organization you're looking to enter a relationship with) you're fiercely loyal and are willing to share all that you have in order to experience a deeper and more truthful connection.

Venus ♀ in Sagittarius ♐ or the 9th House of Purpose

You're a freedom-seeking adventure-ess who loves nothing more than to step off the edge of any zone you deem 'comfy,' directly into the unknown. You need to feel a sense of freedom, even in relationship with others, and it's how you cultivate the most nourishing career – through travel, teaching, and broadcasting your beliefs and knowledge.

To be in relationship with others there must be a promise of growth and expansion to ensure that you stay interested. Ideally, you'll receive a forever-rotating range of possibilities and opportunities – you don't need proof, you just need to feel it, otherwise you'll be quick to swerve any form of commitment. (Especially if people are trying to restrict you, want you to conform, or are tying you down to routines.)

You love to experience the thrills of life, and you're a firm believer in the adage 'fortune favors the bold.' It's this, along with your fun-loving free spirit, that ensures you're guaranteed an invite to every social event and party; other people find your risk-taking lust for life very attractive.

Venus ♀ in Capricorn ♑ or the 10th House of Social Status

Now, you take matters of love and relationships of every kind VERY seriously, preferring to spend quality time (with a heavy emphasis on the word *quality*) getting to know who you might be entering into relationship with rather than jumping straight in.

You're not afraid of hard work and you make money when you take the lead. You're interested in building a strong connection that will create long-lasting relationships and legacy, and you're not easily swayed by big gestures, words of affection, or compliments: You care much more about respect and recognition and whether this project/career/relationship/ friendship is going to be worthwhile. What do they know? What have they accomplished? What do they bring to the relationship?

Basically, entering relationship with you feels very much like being on a VIP list to THE most exclusive of clubs, because if someone does pass the very detailed selection process, they get access to you at your most vulnerable, generous, loveable, and committed.

Venus ♀ in Aquarius ♒ or the 11th House of Friendships

If there was a rulebook to life, you'd be the first to rip it up. You have absolutely no interest in following anyone's rules, and people-pleasing is definitely not on your list of priorities. You actively embrace the unusual and the unconventional and the more shocking the act or experience, the more pleasure you get from it. Some of my favorite women and Wild Roses, Yoko Ono, Gertrude Stein, and Simone de Beauvoir, have this placement and it's clear to see why.

You're a futurist, a visionary who loves to think outside the box, and it's how you're best able to make money. You love for the people you're in relationship with to be that way too. You're not averse to exclusivity when in relationship with others, but you do need to be fascinated, to be challenged, and you thrive when faced with the unexpected.

Venus ♀ in Pisces ♓ or the 12th House of Subconscious

If you had just one mantra, it would be 'I experience my life simply for the poetry of it.' To you, life and love and everything in between is a delicious experience, and you do it all for the poetry, the art, the magic that you experience by living it. From running a bath to eating a juicy peach, there's a natural inclination toward pleasure. Sigh.

It's all about the romance for you in ALL areas of your life, and you have the potential to shape-shift into the dreamiest version of you that's required for any situation. This can be fun, and it comes much easier to you than having to commit. Not because you're incapable of it but mainly because you're quick to feel 'captured' when real life gets a little real life-y, and your first instinct is always to escape. The ideal scenario is to make sure there's always space, in both love and work relationships, to experience the 'poetry' of life, so you don't need to project, shape-shift, or escape.

How does YOUR Venus placement feel to you?

What I've shared here is intended simply to give you a feel for themes and patterns, so that you can then explore on your terms and in your own way. And in true contradictory style, what I've shared here ARE the Venus placements experienced by the thousands of women and clients I've worked with and read for over the years.

Reading their Venus placements in relation to their life experiences has most definitely been a revelatory and a revolutionary codex, for them and for me. If what you read doesn't resonate, there could be other planetary placements that challenge your Venus placement. So, let it be simply a starting point – take what feels right and ignore what doesn't. OK?

Are you a morning star Venus or an evening star Venus?

Don't put your natal/birth chart away just yet because I'd love for us to go even deeper and explore whether you're a morning star or evening star Venus person. I share more about the metaphorical and allegorical significance of Venus's phases in SHE salons 3-5, but here I'll talk specifically about two of her main phases: morning and evening star.

For millennia, many world cultures believed that Venus was two separate planets because they saw a bright planet in the eastern morning sky for seven-ish months and then that would disappear and there'd be a bright planet in the Western evening sky for seven-ish months. It was a hot minute before they realized that this was the SAME PLANET.

You can find out whether you're a morning star Venus or an evening star Venus by locating the placement of Venus in relation to the sun in your natal/birth chart. First, find the symbol for the sun on the zodiac wheel. If you're a *morning star*, Venus will be 'behind' the sun and/or in the previous astrological sign. If you're an *evening star*, Venus will be 'in front' of the sun and/or in the following astrological sign.

NOTE: If your Venus and sun are in the same astrological sign – mine are both in Scorpio – check the degree, because if Venus is FEWER degrees than the sun and closer to the previous astrological sign, it's morning star Venus. And if Venus is MORE degrees than the sun and closer to the following astrological sign, it's evening star Venus. My Venus, in Scorpio, is MORE degrees than the sun and closer to the next astrological sign, Sagittarius, so I'm an evening star Venus.

If you're a morning star Venus

You are SHE who INITIATES. You're likely to be someone who loves to try new things; and someone who values mistake-making and risk-taking and has a can-do attitude. I think of morning star Venus as Wild Rose Joan of Arc, who is a brave leader and ready to make moves.

If you're an evening star Venus

You are SHE who KNOWS. You're likely to be someone who has experienced a LOT and has possibly had what feels like a lifelong dance with the process of death and rebirth.

Therefore, you're much less likely to overreact to situations and are far more capable of cultivating compassion. I think of evening star Venus as Mary Magdalene, who is a medicine keeper, a wise one who is bold and trusts herself.

Again, these aren't intended to be prescriptive – they're simply starting points. As you work WITH the Venus cycle, and experience each of these phases in real time, you'll start to recognize their distinct qualities and flavors and my invitation is for YOU to start witnessing and journaling what they reflect to you about you.

Venus retrograde

Now that you have a flavor of Venus in each astrological sign and house, and you know whether you're a morning star or evening star person, I want to talk about another of Venus's key phases: the retrograde. You've probably heard of a Mercury retrograde – when from our viewpoint on Earth, that planet appears to go backward in its orbit. It's the planetary phenomenon that gets the most PR, mainly because we experience it at least three times a year. However, every planet has a retrograde period, including Venus.

Venus retrogrades every 18ish months, for 40ish days, and it's when she transforms from evening star Venus - bright and visible in the evening sky, and usually the first celestial object we can see as the sun goes down - to morning star Venus, when she's at her brightest, which is just before the sun rises.

In the middle of Venus's retrograde, there's a period of around eight to ten days where Venus is at her closest to Earth but is no longer visible to us in the sky, and that's because she forms a cazimi. A cazimi is an astrological term that refers to a planet that's in close or exact conjunction with the sun and is therefore said to be right 'in the heart' of it. How delicious is that word AND concept?! (We'll talk more about cazimis and Venus in SHE salon 5.)

Yep, the sun and Venus meet at the exact same zodiac point in the sky in an inferior conjunction (a conjunction is when two or more celestial objects come into alignment with each other in the night sky). It's the point where Venus transforms herself from evening star to morning star and begins a brand-new 584-day cycle. For 263 days (roughly nine months) she's morning star Venus; then she enters what I call the 'underworld' phase (more on this later), disappears behind the sun, and becomes evening star Venus for the next nine months of the cycle.

A Venus retrograde is a time to observe your relationships and key themes; and to reassess and heal issues around money, relationships, values, and self-esteem. It can stir up matters of the heart, revealing weak spots and areas for improvement so that we can come OUT of the Venus retrograde with a greater love and respect for ourselves and for others.

The Venus Return

Another key astrological Venus 'moment' is our Venus Return. Each year, Venus returns to the astrological sign that she was in when we were born. Some astrologers consider that to be our Venus Return; however, there's a point every eight years when Venus returns almost exactly to the *degree* that she was at in the sky on the day we were born.

Therefore, since your eighth birthday, you've been having a Venus Return every eight years. As a result, the following years become your significant Venus years – 8, 16, 24, 32, 40, 48, 56, 64, 72, 80, 88, 96, 104 years. And in each of these significant years, Venus holds her mirror up to show you MORE of what wants to be revealed and felt on a deeper level, in terms of YOUR feminine frequency and expression. How that looks and feels will depend on your relationship with the planet, your body, and your frequency.

I spent my 40th birthday and fifth Venus Return in Paris (yes, I LOVE that city!), obsessed with following HER rose lines, and I got a VERY clear message that my siren call, while always nodding to the more mythical and mystical rose line, was to follow MY own rose line. I've since spent a lot of dreamtime revisiting some of those ages when I wasn't aware of my personal Venus cycle and asking to see and witness and feel what wanted to be revealed, and more importantly, honored and revered, at the ages of 8, 16, and 24. I then created a ritual for them so I can embody and integrate them to become MORE of my fullest expression.

Invitation:
Retrospective Venus Return integration

Everything we're doing here is simply to get to know ourselves and all of our parts, so that we're always becoming MORE of who we already are. This opening and acknowledging process is another invitation IN.

What you'll need

Your journal and a pen; a candle; rose oil/rose water; an open heart.

What to do

Start by creating a meditative space where you won't be disturbed. Light your candle, get cozy, and when you're ready, take some beautiful big breaths. Let yourself be present, in your body and start to soften.

Place a little rose oil/water in the palm of your hands and bring them close to your face as you inhale. Let the rose oil/water help your heart to soften, as you come in and come down, into your body, into your heart.

In your own time, set the following intention (you can either say it out loud or write it in your journal):

I invite myself at age (insert age you'd like to call in) at the time of my Venus Return to reveal in the mirror of Venus what I need to know, what wants to be recognized, acknowledged and honored.

Now allow yourself to be open to receive. I open my journal and simply allow what wants to be revealed to be written on the page, but you may receive images, or hear words and phrases.

Of course, if you keep a diary or have photos of yourself at the ages you'd like to return to, refer to those for help and maybe to create a little cosmic nudge. But you definitely don't need them. Setting the intention to connect and receive is enough.

As an example, here's how I approached this process.

- ❖ *At age eight, I got a very clear visual of my grandparents really loving on me with words of affirmation and care; they were tending to me and really encouraging me to express myself. I took that as my Venusian cue to bless my eight-year-old self all the way up with powerful words of love and encouragement every day.*

❧ *At 16, there was a LOT of clearing up to do as I realized that's when I let the external world really impact my internal experience. A lot of my stories about how worthy (or in this case, NOT worthy) of love I was lived here.*

❧ *At 24, I'd become really good at wearing masks, saying the right thing, pleasing and appeasing others. Yet a LOT of shame lived here – I barely recognized myself, so this one took a little more work. I sat and journaled with her for a few hours to find out who she would have been and wanted to be without the masks. There was some deep sadness that she never felt safe to be who she wanted to be. What was revealed is that I had to un-shame myself, my nervous system, so I could create and share from there.*

I did this several times over a few months, and when I was done, I blessed each of these versions of me by placing a dab of rose oil at my heart. I then thanked them and invited what had been revealed to land in my body so that I could honor and revere it through the moves I make, the way I talk to myself, and the stories I now tell. And, more importantly, the life I CHOOSE to live on the daily.

I invite you to do the same or to create your own way to honor and revere the medicine and magic that's revealed to you in this process.

I now very much live IN to these cycles – the Collective Venus cycle and my own personal Venus cycle. They both hold a LOT of medicine for my understanding of how I create more harmony and more alignment with what ACTUALLY matters.

Follow your Wild Rose petaled path

Let Venus be your mirror

Whether it's about your self-worth, love and relationships, your finances, or what it is that you truly value, Venus will reflect it back to you – that's why her astrological symbol is a mirror. So, when you come into a lifelong relationship with Venus, you come into a lifelong relationship with yourself.

Connect to your magnetic frequency

Your natal Venus placement, while NOT diagnostic, is definitely a starting point for exploration as it can offer you intel and support in living in your truest, heart-led expression. (And we ALL want more of THAT, don't we?)

Throw your own notorious NCB salon

Venusian exploration is WAY more fun when shared with friends and loves – make like Natalie Clifford Barney (the notorious NCB) and gather your favorites to compare birth charts and natal Venus placements. (If you want the truth, invite a Scorpio. Just saying.)

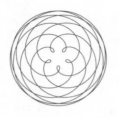

Venus is my
love language.

WILD ROSE SHE SALON

The Venus Cycle

In this salon, we'll look at Venus's revolutions, her phases, and her Wild Rose cosmic dance. Cycles hold the original templates, frequencies, and rhythms for the harmonics of all things and Venus and her cycles (I say cycles plural because she has cycles within cycles) are quite literally the most delicious and harmonic dance.

A Venus cycle revolution – in *all* the ways – happens when the cycle is fully experienced, completed, learned from, metabolized, and alchemized. When we work *with* the cycle and let it support *us* to continually align, refine, and redefine our experience of life with curiosity and endless fascination. When we let it bring heart-led direction to all that we do, and all that we are in the world.

Before we dive into the Venus cycle, let's meet a Wild Rose who's been called the 'rebel queen of the Middle Ages' and the 'Scarlett O'Hara of the 12th century': Eleanor of Aquitaine. Queen of both England and France, Eleanor was one of the most powerful and influential women in medieval Europe. She was known for her intellect, beauty, and assertiveness; and in an age when most people died in their 40s and 50s, she lived to 82.

She defied the societal norms of her times – we already love her for that – and became a trailblazer for women's empowerment as well as a political strategist.

Eleanor's deep love for literature inspired the creation of many works that celebrated Venusian ideals, and she was also THE Creatrix of the 'Court of Love.' Yep, characterized by a brilliant courtly society in which women held the supreme place, the Court of Love (like the Parisian salons that came much later) saw women gather to define the 'rules' of social etiquette, relations, and love and was instrumental in the development of the lyrical poetry tradition of the troubadours.

Now, and here is where it gets SUPER interesting, in his book *Eleanor of Aquitaine*, Jean Markale suggested that the roots of the rituals that were recreated during the Court of Love go all the way back to the great Mother Goddess. It's also said that Eleanor of Aquitaine, like many of the French queens, was a keeper of the Magdalene mysteries, and that beneath the refined poetry of the troubadours, verses of sexual initiation and the Venus cycle were woven. I KNOW! So, what's the fascination with this cycle? Let me tell you.

The Rose of Venus

Over eight years, Venus completes 13 orbits of the sun, and during these eight years, Earth and Venus meet five times. In the process, they create a five-pointed star/five-petalled rose in the cosmos (*see the illustration opposite*). Each star point/rose petal is formed during the Venus retrograde phase of a synodic Venus cycle (a synodic cycle is the relationship that a planet has with the sun; the Venus synodic cycle is 584 days, or roughly 19 months.)

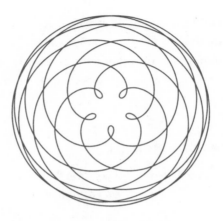

Venus's orbital pattern/the Rose of Venus

The glorious fivefold geometric pattern that Venus makes as she dances with Earth and the sun is known as the Rose of Venus or the Pentagram of Venus (and FYI, it includes the numbers 5, 8, and 13 – five Venus cycles over eight years and 13 trips around the sun – which belong to the Fibonacci sequence that's found throughout all of creation. Magic, right?)

For millennia, the world's cultures were highly attuned to, and aligned with, the Venus cycle. Records of astronomical observations of Venus date back to the 17th century BCE – that's beginning-of-civilization territory right there – to the Venus Tablet of Ammisaduqa created by the Babylonians in Mesopotamia. And in the Americas, the Maya people considered Venus to be the center of the universe, more important even than the sun, and they based their religion and worship on the Venus cycle. This is why, I believe, so many of us today are being called to reconnect with Venus's cycle (and its frequency and the magic it holds).

The Venus cycle is a thing of such beauty, though, that it can make you want to skip over the mechanics of 'how it works' and dive straight into the poetry of it all. Please say that's not just me?! But to be able to fully experience the magic, mythos, and medicine of Venus (and the art and the poetry, troubadour style) it really does help to know 'how it works.' (Even the mechanics are beautiful, I promise.)

The phases of Venus

Now, in case you're like me and you feel that you need to sit with a glossary to grasp some of the astrological terminology around planetary cycles and phases, I'm going to keep this as simple and accessible as possible. Not because we don't/can't/won't understand but simply because when I first took my own lineage of experiential Sky Reading and tried to learn and map Western astrology alongside it, I became overwhelmed very quickly. And while it is beautiful, the Venus cycle is not as straightforward as the moon's cycle and phases, for example, and I'd have loved someone to break it all down for me. So that's what I'm doing in the illustration opposite and brief descriptions of the phases of Venus.

Venus inferior conjunction with the sun/retrograde

Venus's cycle begins during her retrograde phase. Venus is retrograde for approximately 40 days and during this period, she's at her closest to Earth and comes into alignment with the heart of the sun at a cazimi (*see page 76*). It's rebirth time - the death of one cycle and the beginning of another. Yep, Venus meets the sun heart to heart at what's called an inferior conjunction - which is when Venus passes between the sun and Earth. She sounds a claxon, or possibly she strums a harp, which sounds FAR more Venusian, doesn't it? Basically, she declares that a new Venus cycle, in a new astrological sign, has commenced.

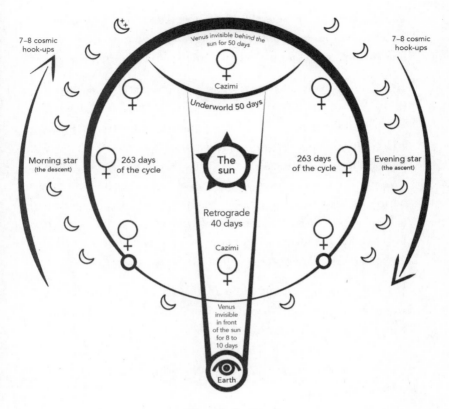

Venus's phases

The retrograde is what I call the reset phase. It's when Venus has completed nine months (263 days) as evening star Venus, which also marks the end of her 19-month synodic cycle. And, like ALL the very best burlesque dancers, she uses this retrograde/reset period to do a full costume change. She assesses what worked (and what didn't) in the last cycle and she tries on outfits before pulling on new stockings, dabbing her favorite oil on the pulse points she wants kissed the most, and putting on a pair of glitzy nipple pasties with tassels that color-coordinate with the astrological sign she's about to cycle through.

Venus prepares for how she wants to be seen, witnessed, and experienced in the world for the new 19-month synodic cycle and the next nine months in her leading role as morning star.

NOTE: Every Venus synodic cycle has an astrological 'theme' that's determined by the astrological sign that Venus is in when she experiences her heliacal rise – her first appearance in the eastern sky. Venus expresses herself, as feminine frequency, through that astrological sign for the entire cycle. For example, if Venus is in the astrological Fire sign of Leo at her heliacal rise, all things Venus – love, money, aesthetics, self-worth, values – will be informed by the themes of Leo (courage, being seen, fun, loyalty, creativity, heart-centered consciousness) for that 19-month (584-day) cycle.

The heliacal rise happens while Venus is still retrograde. It's like a cheeky burlesque toe-poke out from behind the 'sky' curtain; we get a taster of what's to come while still getting to work with the retrograde phase, making any last-minute costume changes around how WE are going to show up and show out during this next Venus cycle.

Venus stations direct/morning star

At the end of the approximately 40-day retrograde/reset, Venus stations direct (moves forward) and is now rising and visible (before sunrise) each morning as the morning star. If you're tuned in to Venus's cycle and/or you've discovered that you're a morning star Venus person (*see page 73*), you may feel that you want to get up earlier, or that you're more inclined to self-start projects and take risks during this period. I highly recommend getting up and greeting Venus, spending time with her in communion each morning, as it's in those early hours that she's at her most potent and powerful.

NOTE: Venus doesn't mess around: 36 days after the heliacal rise, she reaches her 'greatest brilliance' (maximum brightness in the sky) before slowly, over seven-ish months, getting dimmer and lower each morning after seven to eight moon conjunctions (more on these coming up).

Venus superior conjunction with the sun/underworld

At the superior conjunction, Venus meets with the sun once again; she's now at her furthest point from Earth, and it's the peak of the cycle. As she was during the retrograde phase, Venus is absent from the sky, invisible to us behind the glare of the sun (the period varies depending on where you are in the world/ your view of the horizon, but it's usually approximately 50 days). This phase is what I call 'underworld' Venus. It's a time to enter the mystery, the not-known, the void.

Evening star

Venus remains hidden in the sky before she reappears, this time in the west, as the evening star. She will be the brightest and probably the first star you'll see in the evening sky before night falls. This is a much easier phase to track, especially if early mornings are NOT your thing, or you're an evening star Venus person (*find out on page 73*). Tuning in to Venus as the evening star will provide you with a more truth-y experience.

Evening star Venus is wise. She's been to the underworld, and she's no longer a warrior – she's a mother-loving empress who KNOWS herself. Venus spends approximately nine months as evening star. She reaches her maximum brightness in the sky after seven to eight moon conjunctions before entering retrograde when, once again, she disappears from the sky to complete both her nine-month cycle as evening star Venus and now her 19-month synodic cycle in this particular astrological sign to make a rose petal/star point and begin a new one.

Look, this is just a surface-scratch of the many, many moving parts of the Venus cycle, some of which I'm still discovering on the daily. My advice? Don't get caught up in the details, and instead, dive in where your heart is called and let Venus's rhythm guide and support yours.

The Venus rhythm

If you've followed a spiritual path yet still feel pushed and pulled by the nature of the 12-month Roman calendar and digital numbers and alarms, Venus's cycle and her specific cyclical rhythm can become THE most effective nervous-system soother because it both creates *and* harmonizes all things, bringing a sense of rhythm to our lives. The Venus rhythm is essentially the rhythm of the waltz. The waltz is 9/12, while Venus's is a beat out at 8/13; however, she sets a very similar rhythm as she dances with the sun and Earth over a period of eight years.

**INVITATION:
DANCE WITH THE VENUS CYCLE**

I'm sharing my own understanding and revealments of Venus and the Wild Rose codes that I've unlocked over time, but what feels more real and important is that YOU begin your own dance with this Venusian cycle and that you recognize and unlock your own codes and understanding. To do this, listen to songs that are set to the rhythm of the waltz; my playlist includes the following:

- *'La Vie en Rose' – Edith Piaf*

- *'At Last' – Etta James*

- *'The Waltz of the Flowers'* from The Nutcracker, *Tchaikovsky*

- *'Come Away with Me' – Norah Jones*

- *'Moon River' – Andy Williams or Frank Ocean*

- *'Runaway' – The Corrs*

- *'Waltz in the Dark' – Matt Nakoa*

- *'Perfect '– Ed Sheeran*

- *'Iris' – Goo Goo Dolls*

As you listen, trace your finger over the illustration of Venus's orbital pattern, the Rose of Venus, on page 87, and let Venus unlock her Wild Rose codes through you. We all hold them. It's why we're here, in this time and place, to remember them and pull at the threads across lifetimes and timelines and use them as we navigate the bigger cycle of a dying system and the birthing of a new Aquarian age.

NOTE: The more you trust yourself and your body as a vessel for the feminine frequency of Venus, the easier it becomes to witness all the places and spaces she's revealing herself to you – in the books you're called to read, the movies that you're called to watch, the locales you're called to visit. She's unlocking her codes within you and asking you, in the here and now, to weave together the threads, the teachings, and the insights that are being awakened in you to create an act of love in service to What Comes Next.

🌹 Follow your Wild Rose petaled path 🌹

Trace the Wild Rose

On my arm I have a tattoo of the five-petaled Wild Rose that's created in the dance between Venus, the sun, and Earth and sometimes, when I want to connect with Venus, I trace her rhythmic dance with my finger. Obviously, YOU don't have to get it tattooed on your body but do trace Venus's path in the cosmos using the illustration I share on page 87. I've infused it with magic whispers to help you remember and connect with her, too.

It's a phase

The Venus cycle, like the moon's, has phases, and the invitation is to use each of those phases to feel, map, and track your experience as a way to align, refine, and define your experience of life, through your body and through the lens of Venus.

Her rhythm, your rhythm

Venus's rhythm, her dance, holds cues and clues to your rhythm, your dance. If the cycle talk becomes overwhelming, shake off the terms and phrases and instead, put on my playlist (see the Dance with the Venus cycle invitation above) or make your own and simply let her rhythm inform YOUR rhythm. As you move, let your body reveal Venus through you.

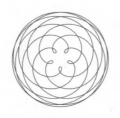

The revolutions
of Venus are what
create personal
revolutions (direct
from the heart).

4

WILD ROSE
SHE SALON

*Myth and Moon Mapping
the Venus Cycle*

In this salon, you'll meet the goddess Inanna, explore the ascent and descent of the planet Venus, and use both the moon and the Inanna myth to map YOUR Venus experience.

As I mentioned earlier, there are stories in most world cultures that map the cycle of Venus and her cosmic dance as she appears, disappears, and reappears in relation to the sun. However, my heart will always take me directly to an ancient Sumerian myth about Inanna, a queen who was considered a divine representation of the planet Venus, and her journey to and return from the underworld, the land of the dead.

A Sumerian poem called 'The Descent of Inanna to the Underworld,' found inscribed on a 7th-century BCE clay tablet from Mesopotamia, recounts one version of the Inanna myth. A mirror of Venus's cycle, it also tells of a time of matriarchal societies and fertility goddess religions and is one of the oldest written-down stories in the world. We'll be looking at and 'mapping' this myth in detail later.

There are other ancient texts about Inanna, including those created by my Wild Rose woman-crush Enheduanna – the ATT (Ancient Triple Threat) – a Mesopotamian poet, high priestess, and princess who was the first named literary author in recorded history. In Sumerian, her name means 'ornament of heaven' and she composed and dedicated 42 devotional temple hymns and three poems to Inanna.

Enheduanna was writing, more than 4,000 years ago, about things that still resonate with us today – insecurities, the creative process, the difficulties of writing a poem (which she equates to giving birth – the woman KNEW). In her hymn 'The Exaltation of Inanna' she portrays Inanna as a powerful goddess of combat and conquest as well as of love, fecundity, and abundance. She refers to her as 'lady of the morning' and 'lady of the evening' because Inanna IS Venus and Venus IS Inanna.

The Inanna-Venus myth

Working with the myth of Inanna's descent to the underworld has created a healing space for me, my own *Carte de Tendre* (map of tenderness) – a framework/container in which to unfold my truth. To come into relationship with myself, with all the versions of me, without judgment.

A place and space where I get to strip them bare and enter IN.

To the underworld.

To the void.

To the place between.

The myth space gives the experience of grief, surrender, letting go, and pain a place to exist that's outside of ourselves. We can then use that space to map it and track it AND we then get to create a pathway back, like Inanna's, for reclamation, harmony, and love.

The fact that the Inanna myth is a beauty-full map of the Venus cycle means that you get to work with it and let it work you in ALL the ways as it brings you home, over and over again with each cycle to become MORE of yourself.

To understand the cycle of Venus, the Sumerians told the story of Inanna, queen of heaven, who ruled over love, fertility, fecundity, sensuality, procreation, and war. There are many modern re-tellings of the myth, but this is mine…

Descent to the underworld

In the time before times, the mountains were young and the sky was clean, and the ibex and the camel walked the desert. The people lived in tents, stone, and cloth. In the land of the living, Inanna (In-arn–ah) and the gods ruled, and in the land of the dead, Inanna's sister Erishkigal (Eh-resh-kee-gal) ruled. In one of those cosmic law things, anyone could enter the land of the living and leave when they wanted to; however, the land of the dead, the underworld, was different. Any being could go to the underworld, but none could return. This was enforced by Erishkigal's servant, Neti, who guarded the gates of the underworld.

There was a situation. There are several ideas about what that *might* have been, with the most popular being that Inanna wanted to attend the funeral of the great Bull of Heaven, Erishkigal's husband. (Now, all these stories are poetic mythos layered with endless meanings, and it's said that the Sumerians used this representation of Erishkigal's husband as the Bull of Heaven to represent the end of the period known as the age of Taurus.) But ultimately, it meant that Inanna *knowingly* made a choice to travel to the underworld to visit her dark sister Erishkigal, queen of the dead.

Realizing that this would be quite the journey, Inanna advised her loyal servant Ninshubur (Nin-shoo-bar) to send for help if she didn't return after three days. And you'd better believe that Inanna put on ALL her royal finery before journeying to the underworld. SO Venusian. As queen she had some pretty bling-y accessories – a golden crown on her head, a lapis lazuli and pearl forehead chain, a lapis necklace, a breastplate, a golden lasso and hip chain, ankle bracelets, and a silky royal robe. BVE – Big Venus Energy.

On hearing of Inanna's journey, Erishkigal insisted that she arrive naked and vulnerable, just like everyone else who entered the land of the dead. Inanna may have been queen of the living, but down there, Erishkigal declared, she would be humbled. (I mean, we can talk about sister wounds ALL day here.)

There were seven gates to move through before entering the underworld, and at each one, Inanna stood and was asked to surrender one of her blingy accessories. Finally, she moved through the seventh gate, and she stood naked before her sister. Again, there's disagreement as to *what* exactly went down, down *there*, but Erishkigal was grieving and, as I'm sure anyone with siblings will testify, fights *can* get gnarly.

Erishkigal let Inanna know: *You're on my territory now. I'm grieving and pissed off. And down here? Things get deathy. Quickly.* Which is how Inanna found herself hung on a meat hook for three days. Over an altar. As a blood sacrifice.

When Inanna failed to return after three days, Ninshubur became concerned about her mistress, so she petitioned various gods to assist with the goddess's rescue. But she only attracted the help of Enki, the god of water and wisdom (they had history, so your woman called in a favor. LOVE that.) Enki offered two representatives, a kurgarra and a galatur, sending them down with the water of life.

After descending, the pair met Erishkigal, who was screaming and lamenting in grief. They held space for her, listening and commiserating, and because of this display of empathy, Erishkigal granted them one wish (genie style). They asked for the body of Inanna, and when they received the corpse, they sprinkled 60 drops of the water of life on Inanna's body and she returned, resurrected.

Slowly, the trio made their way back up through the seven gates, and at each one, Inanna was re-adorned with her accessories as she regained her strength and power and returned to her full glory as queen, forever changed. (This represents the phase when Venus appears at her brightest in the sky.)

Yes, that's my highly simplified version of the Inanna myth, to highlight the connective pieces of *our* exploration together here. As I say, there are many versions of this story and if Inanna feels like *your* key in to working with Venus, my invitation to you is to go find one that sings to your heart. However, I do really recommend reading Diane Wolkstein's book *Inanna*.

Mapping the Inanna-Venus myth

The myth of Inanna's descent to and ascent from the underworld is a Venusian mirror reflection of the 19-month Venus synodic cycle that begins with the planet Venus in her morning star phase. After the retrograde conjunction, as Venus passes between the sun and Earth, she begins what's termed by many as a 'heroine's journey.' It's why the Venus cycle holds so much more potency for those of us who seek something more nourishing and supportive than what the mythologist Joseph Campbell called the 'hero's journey' - the archetypal story template in which the hero goes on an unexpected adventure, learns lessons, acquires knowledge, is transformed, and then returns home in triumph.

The heroine's journey certainly resembles this, but the Venus cycle… well, it's a feminine experience. In the morning star phase of the cycle, representing the outward-facing nature of Venus, like Inanna, like the Fool card in the tarot, the heroine sets off on an adventure.

And I often wonder if Inanna, like so many of the Wild Roses on my Wild Rose path, was a Scorpio. Why? Because her adventure was to the underworld to pay her respects to her sister's husband, but she *really* dressed up for the occasion, wearing all the things that repped her as a queen. Basically, your woman wore FULL ceremonial regalia to get death-y. (LOVE her for that.)

The Venus–moon cosmic hook-ups (CHUs)

Now, during each lunar cycle, Venus and the moon meet in what in astronomical terms is a 'conjunction' (in shamanic astrology, it's a 'gate') and what I call a 'cosmic hook-up,' or CHU.

In the myth, Inanna must pass through seven gates before entering the underworld. And during a 19-month Venus synodic cycle, every month, the planet Venus makes seven or eight conjunctions with a waning (getting smaller) crescent moon as she descends, as morning star, on her way to invisibility from the sky/into the underworld. And these Venus–moon meetings are the cosmic hook-ups (CHUs). Yep, Venus, like Inanna, passes through each of these gates/cosmic hook-ups as she descends toward the horizon.

For seven-ish months, at each cosmic hook-up as Venus descends toward the horizon, you too can map this journey, through your own body, using the seven chakras/energy centers in your body, to willingly choose to experience the descent as a self-initiatory practice. Venus, like Inanna, takes us on what I call a 'Venus SHE quest.' As she makes her descent as the morning star, each cosmic hook-up – the time each month when Venus and the moon are conjunct – represents a descent IN to the body, from the crown chakra to the root chakra, if you're willing.

When Venus becomes invisible in the sky, like Inanna, we too are invited to spend time in the 'underworld.' To complete the Venus synodic cycle, every month, Venus then makes seven or eight conjunctions with a waxing (getting bigger) crescent moon as she ascends as the evening star. Yep, after the descent, and time spent in the underworld, each cosmic hook-up on the Venus SHE quest represents an ascent back up and through the body, from the root chakra to the crown chakra.

While the new and full moons connect us to the lunar feminine and anchor us into our emotions, our unconscious, and our conditioning, the monthly CHUs align us with not only the evolutionary energies of what astrologer Adam Gainsburg, author of *The Light of Venus*, calls the 'Solar Feminine' but also a way to map, experience, and most importantly FEEL Venus through her cycle, via the chakra system, through our bodies.

What I share in relation to this particular exploration – the Venus SHE quest – has been inspired by the groundwork of Daniel Giamario, founder of the School of Shamanic Astrology, and is woven with my own experience and explorations of charting and working intimately with the Venus cycle since 2012.

Shamanic astrology has probably resonated with me more than any other kind of Western astrology, as it not only nods to the ancestors and way-showers in a respectful way but it's also the closest to my own lineage of Sky Reading. (However, as is the case with so much of the Gypsy/Traveller medicine and magic, especially that within my own matriarchal lineage, it's not been recorded in writing but shared and passed down through stories and felt experience. Which is why I'm always sure to name it, and if you ever have a reading with me, you will always experience it first-hand too.)

I'm forever fascinated as to how these maps and ancient-future languages are revealing themselves to us to help us understand this journey and how it's in TOTAL harmony with all that's been and all that will be in this glorious cosmic dance.

The cyclical map of Venus

The first seven Venus–moon conjunctions/CHUs are an opportunity to witness, recognize, and like Inanna, strip yourself of anything and everything that isn't your truest expression as you too descend and enter the 'underworld.' So that as you rise – rooted in the dark – the following Venus–moon conjunctions/CHUs are an opportunity to reclaim and call back our power and magic on your terms.

In the next Wild Rose SHE salon, *Working with the Venus Cycle*, I share rituals and practices to connect you with the seven chakra/energy centers of your body – crown, third eye, throat, heart, solar plexus, sacral, root – at each CHU. Here's the order of the seven CHUs on the descent of Venus, along with the chakra/energy center (and its color and key theme) for each one.

Cosmic hook-ups (CHUs) on the descent of Venus

❋ 1st CHU – Crown chakra; color: violet; key theme: authority/agency/sovereignty; Inanna accessory: golden crown

❋ 2nd CHU – Third eye chakra; color: purple; key theme: perception/inner vision; Inanna accessory: lapis and pearl forehead chain

❋ 3rd CHU – Throat chakra; color: blue; key theme: communication/voice; Inanna accessory: lapis necklace

❋ 4th CHU – Heart chakra; color: green; key theme: compassion/love; Inanna accessory: breastplate

❋ 5th CHU – Solar plexus chakra: color: yellow; key theme: personal power; Inanna accessory: golden lasso/hip chain

❋ 6th CHU – Sacral chakra; color: orange; key theme: sensuality/creativity; Inanna accessory: ankle bracelets

❋ 7th CHU – Root chakra; color: red; key theme: life force/source; Inanna accessory: royal robe

The Inanna myth, the Venus cycle, the astrological sign, the chakra/energy centers in your body, and the rituals and practices I share for each CHU combine to create a spiritual technology that's encoded with many different layers of meanings. I call this the Venus SHE quest and it's a container of both self-revealments and self-initiation. You'll create your own SHE quest in the next SHE salon.

I'm all about connecting with and celebrating the rhythms of the cosmos that support us in restoring the feminine frequency here on Earth. So, through Self Source-ery – which for me is the culmination of the medicine I remember and create through the cycles of my body, the seasons, the moon, and Venus – I've witnessed how I can use my rhythmic intelligence to serve myself AND others and how it's so much easier for me to attune to and align with my truth, my knowing, my real, my siren song.

The descent

When Venus passes through each of the waning crescent moon gates/cosmic hook-ups she disappears beneath the horizon and is no longer visible in the sky. In the myth, this is when Inanna has entered the underworld. She's no longer 'lady of the morning' and she's not yet 'lady of the evening'; she's naked in the dark.

When you arrive at the 'metamorphic underworld' (when Venus moves toward a conjunction with the sun, which means she's invisible behind the sun's glare for approximately 50 days), you 'die' to What's Been Before and all that you thought you were, so you can remember and rebirth wiser and rooted IN your power.

Just as Venus does when she drops below the horizon as the morning star to be reborn as the evening star; just as the moon does when she wanes into the darkness to appear a few days later as a waxing crescent; just as you do, if you bleed, when you move from pre-menstruation into the darkness of menstruation so you can be rebirthed ready for a new cycle of unfolding, SHE/nature/the cosmic g-friend has built-in periods of 'death,' time out for processing, a time for the shadow work to happen. This is where you access what REALLY matters.

In the myth, Inanna descends to the underworld, where she meets her sister Erishkigal, who is its queen. And for us, taking the journey alongside her, this is where we enter the womb-black void. It's here in the depths of the cauldron – our physical womb if we have one, the cosmic womb if we don't – that we're able to meet the dark feminine, SHE of the Dark Matter. To spend those days while Venus is no longer visible in the sky entering into the deep, dark woods, stripped of all we thought we were, looking to reclaim ourselves. The places and spaces where parts of us have been exiled, hidden, suppressed, and repressed.

Our bite.

Our power.

Our courage.

Our knowing.

A remembrance that here, in the dark, is where you/we came from.

I *especially* love the cyclical map of Venus because so many of us avoid the darkness, preferring to stay in the light, make a peace sign and shout 'positive vibes only.' That's great, until an event or situation comes along that takes you out at the knees and you're *not* prepared – physically, mentally, emotionally, spiritually – for how to navigate the dark places.

This cyclical map takes us on a journey that we *choose* to make, a conscious shedding of that which no longer serves us. A release of all the things that restrict us which we 'think' we need, all the places we fight and resist. We retrace Inanna's steps, and we enter the darkness of the underworld and surrender. While in the story Erishkigal hangs her sister on a meat hook, we can take this time – in the darkness of our own womb, in the void of the cosmic womb – to really know ourselves in this place.

Death and rebirth

After passing through the seven gates, Inanna encountered all her egoistic traits, shadow parts, fears, concerns, and uncertainty, all her 'power' was stripped from her, and she was required to die (surrender) to who she believed herself to be. This is the underworld. It's death and rebirth THROUGH surrender.

The gift of the Inanna myth, of the Venus cycle, is that it reminds us that THROUGH surrender, the death initiates a rebirth. It brings us up and through the birthing canal to a more empowered and magical way of being and experiencing life. This has been my BIGGEST teaching from working so intimately with this cycle: Yes, the dark is scary AND it's where we grow our strongest roots. It's where we become aware of what we're most capable of. And most importantly, it's where we truly recognize that in death – both real and metaphorical – we truly remember how to live.

The ascent

Then, just as day follows night, we return. Inanna-Venus meets with the moon, returning back *through* the seven gates in reverse order, and we can map this once again through the seven CHUs; this time, those gates appear at the waxing crescent moons. In the myth, at each gate, Inanna receives back one of her accessories, but *because* of her time in the underworld, and the transformation she experienced, her relationship to those items of power, and the nature of her own power, has been forever transformed. And so, we too get to experience through that ascent the taking back of OUR power, as we rise back up and through the chakras of our body at each CHU.

Here's the order of the CHUs on the ascent of Venus, along with the chakra/energy center (and its color and key theme) for each one.

Cosmic hook-ups (CHUs) on the ascent of Venus

* 7th CHU – Root chakra; color: red; key theme: life force/source; Inanna accessory: royal robe

* 6th CHU – Sacral chakra; color: orange; key theme: sensuality/creativity; Inanna accessory: ankle bracelets

* 5th CHU – Solar plexus chakra: color: yellow; key theme: personal power; Inanna accessory: golden lasso/hip chain

* 4th CHU – Heart chakra; color: green; key theme: compassion/love; Inanna accessory: breastplate

* 3rd CHU – Throat chakra; color: blue; key theme: communication/voice; Inanna accessory: lapis necklace

* 2nd CHU – Third eye chakra; color: purple; key theme: perception/inner vision; Inanna accessory: lapis and pearl forehead chain

* 1st CHU – Crown chakra; color: violet; key theme: authority/agency/sovereignty; Inanna accessory: golden crown

On our ascent – which IS a journey and it's NOT one to be rushed – we must pass back up and through the 'gates,' through the body, through the chakras, from root to crown, claiming, honoring, and revering at each cosmic hook-up between the moon and Venus what was revealed to us in the dark. The evening star phase activates the more receptive nature of Venus as harmonizer and bestower of all the blessings. Likewise, an older, wiser, and initiated Inanna is resurrected, rebirthed, and returns as queen.

However, just as it was for Inanna in the story, you'll find that you don't return from the underworld full of love, light, and all things sugary sweet. No, the light that we bring, when transmuted in the underworld, is stripped back, naked, underneath the skin of it all TRUTH. (Imagine if we were all able to create and share from THAT place!)

NOTE: You'll notice that as Venus descended, stripping herself bare of power to enter the underworld, the moon too was getting smaller, and now as she ascends, taking back her items of power, taking back her own power, the moon is getting bigger. Like I said, everything about the Venus cycle creates THE most delicious harmonics.

Venus retrograde

We then re-enter the period of Venus retrograde and for me, it's here that the ACTUAL initiation happens. You've returned, different to how you left. You've completed your Venus SHE quest (for this cycle at least) and you take the time before the new 19-month synodic cycle begins to rest and digest – to take a full inventory of ALL that's unfolded over that cycle, the entire experience of your very own Venus SHE quest.

The retrograde is YOUR opportunity to be in ceremony with it ALL before you begin a new revolution of the cycle. We do this together in the SHE Power Collective every Venus retrograde and it's really powerful.

To recap, during her 19-month synodic cycle, Venus makes seven conjunctions/CHUs with a waning crescent moon as she descends as morning star on her way to invisibility/the underworld. And she then makes seven conjunctions with a waxing crescent moon (as she climbs toward her maximum brightness as evening star). Join us at the SHE Power Collective, where we do this together and I share in real time, which removes a LOT of the guesswork and research.

The 8th cosmic hook-up

Now, while it's *always* seven Venus and moon conjunctions (CHUs) because that's the Venus math, sometimes there may be a cycle where we experience an 8th cosmic hook-up either side. (As I've said, the Venus cycle isn't always straightforward – and why SHOULD she be? She's anything *but* linear). This is why, when we explore the cycle using the chakra system through the body, it isn't a 'perfect' fit. However, and this is the important bit, it is a *harmonic* fit and Venus is ALL about the harmonics. In the SHE Power Collective, if we DO experience an 8th CHU, we feel into it as our energetics – our vibration and our frequency.

You always have a choice

My journey with Venus and Inanna began in the darkness and grief of my mumma's terminal diagnosis. And as with every heroine's journey, it's rare that the descent from power and safety is ever voluntary. In fact, a rapid descent often occurs on this particular path when someone who the journey-taker – the heroine – loves is taken from them. The Venus cycle, however, offers us a map, an opportunity to actively *choose* to enter in. So that when we inevitably *do* find ourselves in the darkness, and we will, we KNOW it.

We know who we are there.

We no longer fear it.

We know what's possible there AND we also know that we can, and that we do, return.

Follow your Wild Rose petaled path

Dare to go there

In Western society, we have few rituals or support for the phases of dying, death, and grief, yet the descent offers an opportunity to choose, like Inanna, to descend. To enter the underworld knowingly and gain intel, cues, and clues as to how to REALLY LIVE.

Root to rise

When you've dared to enter the underworld, and stayed there in the dark, you grow strong roots. You don't build your home there, but you do remain connected to a deep and ancient feminine wisdom as you rise, rooted and ready to thrive.

Own your experience

It sometimes seems much easier to let life happen to you, to deal with the inevitabilities of life as and when they occur. However, when you map and track your experience using Venus and her connections to the moon and mythos as a sacred container, like Inanna, you can use what's revealed to Self Source and dream into being YOUR experience. YOU, on YOUR terms.

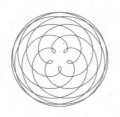

Deeply descend.
Root, source,
then rise.
Steady and wise.
Remembering how
to be fully alive.

5

WILD ROSE SHE SALON

*Working with
the Venus Cycle*

In this salon, we'll work with the Venus cycle as a felt and embodied ritual and ceremony. Mapping the Inanna-Venus myth, the moon, and the Venus cycle gives us a support tool to help us explore and make meaning of our experience called 'This Life.' My husband, the Viking, and I both lean heavily into the practice of mapping and tracking in ALL of our work. And it's how I'm really able to explore MY Wild Rose path, MY experience; to get curious as to *why* I feel the way I do and *how* I'm able to stay present and IN my body so that I can witness and recognize if and when I need to course correct.

When I map and track my experience of the Venus cycle, I do it predominantly through my feels. I know some people like science and facts, but I won't lie, I have *very* little interest in those – mainly because they're determined by someone else's experience, not mine. I'm very much a feeler and experiencer of life, and it's by FEELING my way through the Venus cycle, as an experience IN MY BODY, that I remember while this is definitely a path without 'certainty,' I *am* able to return 'home,' to become more of myself and activate and claim my Wild Rose medicine, the medicine of my heart.

The felt experience of life-living

Wild Rose Josephine Baker was the epitome of a woman IN HER BODY, and she's very much a guide-ess for us all in the FELT experience of life-living. The world-famous dancer, singer, enchantress, activist, and icon ran away from home at the age of 13 to join a travelling show. She arrived in Paris from the US in the mid-1920s, after World War I, and it was said by many at the time that she taught everyone how to live again.

Josephine defied all the beauty ideals of the age and dared to create her own. She used her drive, determination, sensuality, skills, and talents to captivate audiences, ensuring that on both stage and screen she stole EVERY SINGLE SCENE.

Josephine was smart – she knew that, at a time when the USA wasn't ready to accept erotic performances like hers, the city of Paris would welcome her; she re-appropriated Europeans' colonial characterizations of the Black body and made them fall in love with her. Author Ernest Hemingway described her as 'the most sensational woman anybody ever saw.'

She was known as the 'Ebony Venus,' the 'Black pearl,' and the 'jazz Cleopatra,' and she was more than OK with that because she *knew* who she was – a one-woman extravaganza. She slept with both men and women and had a pet cheetah that she'd walk in the streets of Montmartre wearing a collar of diamonds.

Later in her life, Josephine was an agent for the French Resistance during World War II; a civil rights activist (in 1963, she was the only woman to speak alongside Martin Luther King Jr. at the March on Washington); and mumma to an adopted family of 12 children from all over the world. She was a force, and in true Wild Rose style, she also owned Marie Antoinette's bed. Clearly, Wild Rose knows Wild Rose. Her funeral? It was held in La Madeleine Church in Paris. (Of course it was.)

Josephine Baker is also one of the main inspirations for a modern-day Wild Rose: the world-renowned burlesque icon Perle Noire, whose on-stage performances are both mesmerizing and a fully felt spiritual experience. Watching her perform is like watching the Goddess incarnate. In fact, it's not *like* watching the Goddess – you ARE watching the Goddess.

I love to dance and perform burlesque, but it wasn't until I saw Perle in the same line-up as burlesque queen of the red-lip Dita Von Teese, dressed as Queen Nefertiti, that I remembered why I've never been quite able to shake – literally – my previous lives as a temple priestess. I wasn't mean to. Perle taught me that it was holy as fuck to embody the Goddess and to dance and move my body in devotion to her. Not to please others – although, sure, I've no doubt it does do that – but as a ritual to activate source power: healing, magnetic, and regenerative magic.

We dance the dance of our rhythmic intelligence and in the dance, I become more me, you become more you, and we become more WE.

Connecting with Venus through the body

It can be oh-so-easy to outsource our growth, joy, pleasure, and self-revealment, especially if we feel like we don't know what it is that we want and need. And yet, for me, connecting with the rhythm and cycle of Venus has become a container within which I can crack my own codes, and it really allows me to feel and trust what it is I want and need.

The Venus cycle is HOW I've become embodied. I've been working intimately with my body and its rhythmic intelligence in relationship with the cycles of the cosmos for many years, but since really getting to know myself in the reflection of Venus's mirror – feeling her cycle and her themes THROUGH my body – I've realized my power truly lies in my choices; how I've been able to build a relationship of love, care, and Self Source-ery with and for myself.

I've learned how to tend to and nourish my body and my spirit. But not with a carbon-copy descriptive and prescriptive 'system.' With each 19-month Venus cycle we're offered a 'structure' that's both nourishing and supportive – a way in, a way through, *and* a way out. And yes, while I've shared with you some of the ways in which the cycle *can* be mapped, I love that it isn't FULLY mappable – which I KNOW will send the detail freaks super crazy.

It's not certain because it's a path of mysteries, keys, and codes and these mysteries, keys, and codes become 'known' when you loosen your grip on needing them to make 'sense.' Instead, they need to *be* sensed. THIS is the way of the feminine.

When I shared the moon and menstrual maps in my book *Code Red*, so many readers wanted, *needed*, their menstrual cycle to 'fit.' They wanted, *needed*, their moods and experiences to be a replica of the examples I'd shared. And when they didn't fit – because they wouldn't, as each of our experiences is entirely unique – they would automatically think that they were doing something wrong. This is because the societal programming has taught us, women especially, to follow rules (when rules are arbitrary) and to think that we're 'wrong' or 'broken' if our experience is somehow different to other people's. NOT TRUE.

It's why I call what I share maps. Whether they relate to menstrual cycles, the moon, or in this case, Venus, they're supportive way-showers with touch points and areas of interest to explore and get curious about. Of course, life inevitably has seasons/times/moments of darkness and despair, and what I love most about the Venus cycle is that it has a period of built-in darkness. It literally plunges you into your own darkness and it's here that you get to choose.

Now, as you know, I'm big on us choosing, taking responsibility for our lived experience, because when those moments/situations come along that we *haven't* chosen, we have the tools. We KNOW how to see in the dark, and we're prepped to navigate it. So, we come down into the body, descending, and at each chakra/cosmic hook-up stripping, unravelling, and revealing ourselves to ourselves and letting go of what's no longer needed and required. We come down into the void, the womb of infinite possibility, and we meet Ma of the Dark Matter, where we recognize and realize what it is that ACTUALLY matters.

And while it CAN feel like despair, it's actually the very best kind of filter, because it means that we can then ascend, with power, reclaiming at each chakra/cosmic hook-up what it is that ACTUALLY matters. Not what we *think* we need. We're without the societal, familial, and cultural programs and conditions, and, because of the nature of being human, there's a likelihood that there will be times when we forget, so we get to experience *another* 19-month Venus cycle, this time with a different astrological theme, with a different quality and flavor of Venus magic and medicine for us to receive and experience. In this way, we deepen and harmonize our relationship with ourselves. It's REALLY BLOODY GORGEOUS. And in doing this, we let MORE of ourselves come online and we really allow ourselves to let what matters – the Venusian qualities of creativity, joy, beauty, and pleasure – be REALLY experienced and FULLY savored. Sigh.

Now, all this can feel very out of step with a world that wants you to hate on yourself and be fretful of everything, and yet there WILL be a freedom. You'll be liberated and much less susceptible to the societal spells. Of course, you can still partake in the buffet of consumerism and capitalism, but it'll be on YOUR terms as you'll be rooted in your truth and your felt, deep, and magnetic feminine knowing.

The IN.YOUR.BODY.MENT Venus SHE quest

The Venus SHE quest is the practice that I've been sharing and tweaking every Venus cycle with the SHE Power Collective as a 'map of possibility' for us to create our own adventure, our own *Carte de Tendre*, our own reality *with* Venus. I provide key marker points and then you, as the visionary, oracle, SHE quester, take those and create your own experience, unlock your own Venus codes, as you explore YOUR Wild Rose path.

NOTE: You don't NEED to follow the Venus cycle to explore YOUR Wild Rose path. You're already traversing the landscape – you wouldn't be here if you weren't. But what I will say is that this cycle has become a way for me to keep returning, over and over, to myself. A heart mapping of what I know to be true (yet forever need reminding of); that I'm my own living mystery school; that I hold the keys and codes for both death and rebirth; and that I'm perpetually becoming, unfolding, and unfurling, one Wild Rose petal at a time. So, y'know, I *do* recommend it. *Wink.*

Look, the astrology might not be your thing, or the Venus mythos might not resonate with you. I get it. What I've found is that connecting with the Venus cycle, in the way that I'm about to share, deepens our self-trust. Even if you're not so interested in the chakra system, simply bringing your attention to those areas of your body in relationship to the Venus experience and frequency WILL bring you into connection with her THROUGH your body.

Having the opportunity to give a nod and a wink to Venus at her cosmic hook-ups with the waning moon on the descent – having that metaphorical time in the underworld to willingly enter the darkness (even if it's just a 10-minute daily meditation in the dark) – and then mapping the ascent, the returning, up through the cosmic hook-ups with the waxing moon and back into the retrograde period for integration, *is* self-initiation. Over and over again, with each and every cycle, into our body, into our own mystery school, into our own remembered magic and onto our own Wild Rose path.

You *can* start your Venus SHE quest at any point in the Venus cycle. Look up where Venus is in her cycle right now as you're reading this – you can either search for this online or join us in the SHE Power Collective (www.lisalister.com/the-she-power-collective). Knowing where Venus is, what phase she's currently traversing, will give you a feel for *your* current landing point. (Remember, there are NO coincidences, so where Venus currently is in her cycle WILL have significance to your life. I promise. Even if at first glance it isn't clear what that is.)

Personally, though, I feel that we receive the most medicine through experiencing the *entire* 19-month synodic cycle, from retrograde through to retrograde, and that's the map I share in this salon. It's important that this does *not* become yet another thing to *do*, though, because it's definitely not that. If you let it, it can become a devotional practice of self-discovery and

Self Source-ery, of deepening your wisdom and knowing, of returning to the feminine magic of the times when we lived our entire mother-loving lives as a rhythmic ceremony.

Make the quest your own

Now, if you already chart, track, and map your menstrual cycle (if you have one) and/or the moon cycle, the Venus SHE quest can be a delicious Venusian-infused add-on to that experience. Since I've been mapping mine in accordance with my menstrual cycle and the moon, the synchronicities and magic that's unfurled has become *my* Self Source-ery.

Or it might be that for a 19-month Venus cycle, this is the *only* thing you map. I know lots of people who, once they've discovered the Venus cycle and the monthly CHUs no longer feel called to pay attention to the new and full moons and instead, plan their rituals and meditations around the cosmic hook-ups. It's a powerful way to work with your body and the Venus cycle and activate your magic, oracular insight, and creativity.

You can make each CHU a whole big and beautiful ceremonial affair. You can dance with the energy and tune in to the frequency of how Venus makes herself known through each chakra/energy center of your body. Or you can take your journal for a date in nature and riff with a prompt or make a cup of your favorite libation and sit with Venus and the moon in an oracular meditation each month and riff on what you receive. There's NO right way to do this, only YOUR way. Let what I share simply be a guide, OK?

Saying that though, if you're called, I do recommend traversing the Venus SHE quest in community with other people, as you learn so much from each other's experiences. There's no one person who holds this wisdom or *teaches* you – we each have our own mystery school teachings INSIDE us and it's through these Venus SHE quests that we unlock those codes; and we might hold codes for others too, so while the quest is always your own, the medicine discovered is most definitely to be shared.

Call back your magnetic source power

It's THROUGH the Venus cycle that we can cultivate our power, magic, and innate feminine wisdom. (Yep, the kind that's been discredited, defamed, and demonized – y'know, the VERY BEST kind.) It's rooted deep in the dark and then blooms like the *wildest* of roses.

Now, the chances are that, no matter how much 'spiritual work' you've been doing on yourself, you may have become a bit leaky energetically. This usually happens when our boundaries aren't defined and strong; when we abandon ourselves to please others and/or we actively choose to stay small because we don't want to be *too* bright, *too* attractive, *too* seen. (Because there's a strong possibility that we've experienced, in this lifetime and/ or past lives, that when we *are* visible, attractive, and seen, our energy IS big, and we DO attract attention. And if we're not ready, or don't have the capacity to hold it, this can cause overwhelm, discomfort, and pain to our body and being.)

So, we can work with the Venus SHE quest to get VERY intentional. We can use it as a way to build a relationship of trust with our body and to grow strong roots. So that when we DO call back, restore, and recalibrate our power, magic, and innate feminine wisdom from time and space, it returns to nourished and fecund terrain – our body – where it has the capacity to grow and expand. Because Venus reflects to us the Self Source-ery we require (and that will be different for each of us) so that we can take radical responsibility for holding, maintaining, cultivating, and strengthening our magic, power, and innate feminine wisdom. Our magnetic source power – the creative power that's *necessary* for us to birth What Comes Next.

The Venus cycle descent is about releasing and letting go of all the things/obstacles/situations/patterns that stop you from TRUSTING your oracular wisdom. Your inner guidance, your belly and bone-deep gnostic knowing. It invites you to, like Inanna, release, de-armor, and soften so that you enter the underworld naked of all the 'things' – material/ego/labels/judgment/stories. The more that's released, the more space and capacity becomes available to us as we enter the underworld. It's here where we can start to trust our own innate wisdom and true essential self. We learn to see in the dark, strengthen our oracular sight, and come to our senses. So that on the ascent, we rise rooted and strong and are able to call back, reclaim, and more importantly, retain and maintain, our power and magic.

Prep for the SHE quest

1. First, know YOUR Venus placement – if you haven't done so already, take a look at where Venus is in your natal/birth chart (*see page 60*) That's YOUR *lifelong* Venus astrological theme – the lens through which the feminine expresses itself in YOU.

2. Next, search online to find out the astrological 'theme' of the *current* Venus synodic cycle. For example, if Venus was in the Fire sign Leo at the heliacal rise of the current cycle, Leo will be the lens through which Venus expresses herself, setting the astrological theme for that entire 19-month synodic cycle. (*To find out how Venus expresses herself in each astrological sign, see pages 63–73*).

3. During Venus's morning star and evening star phases,
    which last around 263 days, each cosmic hook-up (Venus-
    moon conjunction) will occur in a different astrological sign.
    I recommend using a good astrology app, such as Time
    Passages, that will give you a daily astrological forecast. (Or
    join the SHE Power Collective, where I share in real time,
    which removes a LOT of the guesswork and research.)

What you'll need

* **A journal and pen** I don't need ANY excuse to buy stationery,
  but having a journal that you dedicate specifically to your felt
  experience of and with the Venus cycle not only becomes a
  delicious self-devotional, but it also acts as YOUR *Carte de
  Tendre* (map of tenderness), charting YOUR Wild Rose path.
  I also have a fancy fountain pen that's embossed with roses
  and uses red ink that smells of red roses – I KNOW!

* **A mirror** This can be your bathroom mirror; or one of those
  gorgeous, elaborate handheld mirrors that Victorian women
  kept on their bedside table (I've always wanted one of
  those); or a compact mirror that you keep in a gorgeous case
  specifically for rituals. I've designed a compact mirror for this
  purpose, and it's available from www.lisalister.com/shop

* **Altar pieces** This one's up to you. If you wish, you can make a
  Venus altar like the one I share on page 26, or you can have
  one set up in your home that you tend to each Friday (Venus
  day) or at which you light a candle on every cosmic hook-up.
  It can be as basic or as fancy as you wish, but let it include
  the Venusian talismanic items that call to YOU. A shell, pearls,
  a pretty mirror, dried rose petals, a rose-oil-infused candle –
  you choose.

In my book *Code Red*, I suggest making a menstrual cycle box in which you gather all the things you like to experience to honor your bleed days, and it might be fun for you to create something similar for the Venus cycle. You may use it every Friday or you may keep it for the moon-thly CHUs. Whatever you decide, keep all the things you love and will want to use in one place. Maybe you have a gorgeous bag in pink or green, the colors of Venus, or maybe you wrap your oracle cards in a scarf that's decorated beauty-fully. Yes, Venus is HEAVY on the aesthetics, but ultimately, it's what feels beauty-full to YOU.

Things to do at the CHUs (cosmic hook-ups)

For each of the seven or eight monthly cosmic hook-ups on both the descent and the ascent, I've provided the following info/rituals/practices/heart riff prompts to help you connect with the chakra/energy center of your body. Our chakras can hold the key to a profound sense of well-being, self-discovery, and healing. When we bring our attention to them and activate them in cocreation with Venusian harmonics, we can unlock a deeper connection to the body, mind, and spirit.

You'll also use the astrological sign in which the CHU occurs that month to journal and heart riff on what you need to take back and really honor, revere, and create ceremony WITH that chakra/energy center (more on that coming up).

Mirror work practice

As I've worked with the Venus cycle, mirror work has become my most treasured practice. Venus's astrological symbol is a mirror, and a mirror is also one of the accessories that Inanna relinquishes (and then reclaims) in the myth. AND mirror work was the signature technique of author, teacher, publisher and one of my all-time favorite inspiring women, Louise Hay (who was most definitely a Wild Rose) for improving your relationship with yourself.

For the cosmic hook-ups on both the ascent and descent, I've shared a mirror practice in which you look at yourself, your reflection, in the mirror, place a hand on your heart and *activate* and *affirm* a positive and supportive statement by repeating it out loud to yourself. I believe that the words we speak are spells. Spoken invocations to bring dreams, ideas, and possibilities into manifest. So, if, like me, you've experienced difficulties when speaking out loud or sharing your voice and truth in the world, use the activate and affirm statement that I share as a practice.

NOTE: Sitting in front of a mirror and repeating positive words about yourself directly at your own reflection can bring up STUFF. However, activating and affirming frequencies IN our body, to support what it is we already know, deep down in our bones and belly, but DEFFO need reminding of daily, can *really* help. If you're like me and have sometimes rolled your eyes at what on the outside seem like 'spirituality lite' practices, what I've found is that the simpler you keep it, the more profound it becomes. Because we really DO forget.

So, for the 'activate and affirm' statement for each CHU I invite you to take some deep breaths, allow your body to soften, and be open to remember and receive the activation as you repeat it three times: the first time to *hear* and *feel* it resonate in your voice through your body; the second time to *activate* it in every cell of your body and being; the third time to *affirm* it in every cell of your body and being.

Now, I call it an activation because these words WILL make you feel a certain way. If you're into it, they'll allow you to remember and feel it more deeply. If you're cynically side-eyeing it/ overthinking, SOMETHING will be activated in you in order for the cynicism/overthinking to even occur. So THAT becomes something to witness as you repeat the statement three times anyway. The intention, the resonance, and vibration of you repeating and affirming the activation WILL work because… it's MAGIC. Ha!

Heart riff prompts

Look, you don't need me to tell you how to journal, and you don't need me to provide you with journal prompts either. Which is why I invite you to consider what I share here as an opportunity to take some deep breaths, come into connection with the chakra/ energy center of the cosmic hook-up, bring your attention to your heart, and then let your heart riff with the question offered as a prompt.

Because these heart riff prompts aren't *just* questions. If you let them, they'll also be psyche-prods. An opportunity to get out of your own way, to stop 'thinking' and instead, drop IN to your body to explore, wander, and get curious about what wants to be revealed, through YOU, in the spaces between each cosmic hook-up during Venus's descent and ascent.

Self Source-ery

Here, I share a nudge of love for you to FEEL into what's required to support and nourish your exploration for the time between each CHU. I call this Self Source-ery – with a heavy emphasis on *source* because it fortifies and strengthens. It supports us to cultivate patience and the ability to listen to our bodies; to come to our senses, to trust our instincts, and to remember our magic in a world that does NOT want us to do that and is not set up in ANY way for us to do that. Remember that this is YOUR Venus SHE quest, so, part of activating and aligning with YOUR rhythmic intelligence is to create what works for you.

NOTE: Self Source-ery is NOT about the fancy things, although it definitely can be. It's about the cultivation of practices that light us and lift us all the way up, that nourish and satiate us. So, make small moves. Work within your budget, your energy range, and with what's accessible to you.

Self-care in ANY form can feel like 'bypassing,' but that's HOW society has been set up – to MAKE us feel guilty and/or selfish for tending to and caring about ourselves; for nurturing and mothering ourselves THROUGH a situation, rather than just BLOODY GETTING ON WITH IT REGARDLESS. Working with the rhythmic intelligence of Venus, creating our own Self Source-ery through ritual and ceremony, supports us ALL to come into harmony with that.

Create your Venus SHE quest

Okay, let's work through the 19-month Venus synodic cycle from retrograde to retrograde.

Phase: Venus retrograde

The Venus cycle begins during the retrograde phase. Now, if I had my way, during the retrograde phase, we'd all get to recline on a chaise longue, eat cake and sip rosehip tea while we really integrate the medicine and magic of the previous 19 months. Because essentially, this is what a retrograde is for: to RE-visit, RE-integrate, RE-assess all that's unfolded and unfurled for you.

There are three key phases to the retrograde; we experience it as before, during, and after a cazimi (when Venus is 'in the heart' of the sun – *see page 76*): before cazimi (BC); the cazimi (TC); and after cazimi (AC). Venus retrograde is when Venus transforms from evening star to morning star: It's when she's most alchemical.

Before cazimi (BC)

This is the time to acknowledge, integrate, and alchemize the last 19 months so that we're prepared for the journey ahead. We need to recognize that an upleveling cosmic glow-up has occurred (and is still in process). By this, I don't mean we've got 'better' than others, but we WILL have grown. There will have been growing pains (and possibly some resistance to that too.) We're shedding old stories, old beliefs, old narratives (and some of us will be grieving those, and it's OK to do that, y'know.)

We're initiating ourselves, and while some of us feel like we know the next step and are eager to move forward, others are feeling VERY unstable and insecure as we wait for new skin to grow before we can move ahead. And that's what THIS part of the Venus retrograde phase is for: to allow our system time to adapt, to fully arrive in its wholeness of who we are, right now, in this moment.

We NEED this time. Many of us have experienced feeling unsafe in our body, in our environment, so it's important to always take the time to land, to be IN your body and to find safe space amid the ever-changing experience. Then, as Venus moves toward the heart of the sun at the cazimi (TC) you MAY feel yourself turn toward your own heart as you too enter the heart of your sun. As above, so below.

The sun represents our sense of self, our identity, who we are. Venus represents our worth, our values, what we love. So, as you move toward the cazimi, check in with YOUR growling desire belly.

What are YOU ravenous for right now? What does your heart TRULY long and yearn for?

Now, the big thing I want to flag up is that in this phase of integration it can be REALLY easy and tempting to find yourself comparing your experience to that of others. But remember: NOTHING compares to you. (Listen to this song. The Sinéad O'Connor version. Cry if you need to. It helps.) And this period is one of inner reflection, so if you recognize that you're seeing someone else's experience and comparing yours to theirs, take a deep breath, place a hand on your heart and return home.

This process is about YOU. You're forever becoming, right? Let it BE alchemical. Let it reveal MORE of your real. Let it reveal MORE of your truth. And when you recognize comparisons, and the old stories and beliefs show up, thank them. And then put them in the alchemical cauldron to reveal MORE of who you REALLY are underneath them. If you're called, write down and heart riff on the following: all your current fears. All the lessons and wisdom that have unfolded for you in the last 19 months.

The cazimi (TC)

Venus enters the heart of the sun at the cazimi. The sun will fill Venus all the way up with information and intel from its heart and it will filter through the heart lens of Venus, directly into YOUR heart. YOU are a Creatrix. So, open yourself as a channel of celebration, a channel of intel, keys and codes and then slow down to receive and digest. This is a death AND it's a rebirth.

NOTE: At the last Venus retrograde, I really grappled with my people-pleaser. I LOVED my people-pleaser; everyone responded so well to her and when they loved her, it 'felt' like they loved me. And it's THAT feeling and sensation that I was grieving, while knowing that she absolutely, positively could no longer live here.

INVITATION – BREATHE AND RECEIVE

The main thing I do on a TC is a simple practice to create the space to receive and then, more importantly, be able to hold what it is I receive. First, find a soundtrack that you like; I put 'I Love You' by Za Rah Kumara on repeat and set a timer for 20 minutes. Not essential, but super nourishing and supportive. You could also make a cup of heart-opening cacao with added rose water, again not essential, but it will offer a lil extra heart soothing.

1. *Find a comfy position, either seated or standing, and take a few intentional sips of cacao, some nice easy breaths in and out, and let yourself land in your body. Then bring your attention to your pelvic bowl, your cauldron of creative power, and start to stir it by moving your hips in a circular motion. There's no right way to do this – we're simply bringing our attention to our pelvic bowl and we're creating circles with it in one direction and then when it feels good, changing direction. Do this to your soundtrack for three to five minutes.*

2. *When you feel comfy and IN your body, you're going to take a conscious breath in through the nose – let the breath come all the way in – and pull it down past your heart, past your belly, and into your cauldron of creative power, your medicine bowl. Right down to your base, your root, where your pythoness resides.*

3. Hold that breath there and as you release it, really slowly through the nose, see if you can keep your attention, and the energetics, IN your cauldron, at your root. That's it. Don't tense your body to 'hold' it, simply let it be present there.

4. We breathe in through the nose, pull the in-breath all the way down, hold it there, and then we release the breath back out through the nose. But we hold the energy that it's created IN our cauldron. I do this stage for 11 minutes, but you can do it for three, or for however long feels good to you.

5. You can turn this practice into a beauty-full ritual by taking a bath or shower beforehand; soak in rose oil, drink cacao or blue-lotus or rose tea, anoint your pulse points with jasmine or rose oil, set up an altar space, put a picture of you on it, and add some shells or any other talismanic items that you associate with Venus.

6. When you're ready, anoint a candle with rose oil and light it. Wrap yourself in your favorite fabrics or do it naked. Stir your cauldron and then settle in to your breath and build the energy IN your pelvic bowl. Declare, **I am open to receive**, and then be prepared to listen.

7. Like Venus, you too are a magnetic vessel, so let Venus, in the heart of the sun, transmit and activate YOUR wisdom. You can journal, heart riff, and draw, but ultimately, let yourself be as quiet as possible to hear and receive what it is you NEED. It might be in words, but it's rarely intellectual, so I suspect it will be more of a felt transmission, body responses – make space for them.

8. Lift up your heart, recognize and give thanks for the past 19 months and allow your heart to now be magnetized toward the creativity, joy, love, and magic that is truly befitting who you are.

The cazimi is a magical and mystical place and space in time to reset. Let whatever you do feel like a ritual of receiving the most delicious warm, runny honey into your entire being, loaded with codes and cues to guide you in the direction of your desires, needs and pleasure.

After cazimi (AC)

A new cycle has begun. Yes, she's morning star Venus AND she's still retrograde, so know that she/you/we are in process (FOREVER in process. Like the burlesque dancer, she/you/we have made the costume change from evening to morning star but before she/you/we go direct, we're practicing our moves, we're trying out the nipple pasties and sparkles to work out which ones we prefer.) This is the rebirth; only we're not quite out of the birth canal yet, so we'll keep witnessing the 'old' ways and patterns that still want and need to be alchemized.

Yes, choices can be made in a heartbeat, and I'm pretty sure that many of us have quantum time-leaping abilities that we're within moments of mistress-ing, but until then, we can use the AC phase of Venus retrograde to really RE-examine and RE-view how we are in relationship with both ourselves and others. So that we're then able to RE-commit to the things that ACTUALLY matter as we prepare for the new cycle. And as we DO prepare, like Inanna, you'd better believe we're putting on our finest queenly bling and regalia.

Final notes for the retrograde phase

Get intentional. Venus is a harmonizer, so while yes, this *is* a phase for introspection, don't get stuck there; use it as an opportunity to get to know and fully understand your needs so that you can effectively tend to yourself and Self Source during this time.

Ask yourself:

* What conditions and relationships do I need to feel worthy and loved?

* What and who is real and important to me?

* How do I want to relate to and with myself AND others?

* What do I want to give MORE space to in my heart and life?

This is NOT a time to start anything new; this is an 'I'm figuring it out' phase. Venus retrograde is known as a time when people make 'interesting' choices, especially in terms of haircuts, appearance, and hooking up in some way with past relationships – with lovers, friends, work colleagues. Loves, MAKE. NO. SUDDEN. MOVES. For sure, reflect on those things, but this is a period of alignment, so let Venus fill you up and create WITH her.

Phase: morning star Venus/the descent

As Venus makes her monthly cosmic hook-ups with the waning crescent moon, we too descend, and on the way, we explore our sense of independence, agency, and self-sovereignty, tuning in and listening deeply to our intuition and body wisdom. And, like Dorothy on the Yellow Brick Road in *The Wizard of Oz*, like anyone who menstruates experiences in the pre-ovulation phase of their cycle, this is a time to take risks, to make mistakes, to have experiences and to use them to notice what is and what is NOT in tune with our hearts.

Your heart is ALWAYS your Venusian compass, and the CHUs act as a moon-thly check in WITH yourself to explore what's truly, authentically you and to let go of what no longer aligns with your truthiest of truths. (Because THROUGH this cycle, you get ruthless about your heart truth. NOT the 'truth' you're *told* to believe. No, the truth that *actually* matters: YOUR heart's truth.)

Morning star Venus CHU steps

1. Each cosmic hook-up will occur in a different astrological sign during a waning (growing smaller) crescent moon. Consult your preferred astrological app for a daily astrological forecast. However, each CHU will occur in the same chakra order, descending from top to bottom, from crown to root, through the seven chakra/energy centers. At each one, I invite you to create a 20-minute ritual/time-out-of-time to connect IN.

   Twenty minutes is one third of an hour, which represents the three days that Inanna was hung on a meat hook in the underworld. (I usually do much longer, but I don't have children, and I appreciate that people's lives are busy, so make it work for you.) It's this devotional reverence to yourself, to the rhythms of Venus, to your cyclical and rhythmic intelligence, to the descent, that provides the Self Source-ery – the medicine that YOU cultivate and cocreate in alignment with what it is you reveal and uncover here.

2. Tune in with the chakra/energy center. Locate it on your body – place a hand there if it helps – bring your attention to that area and breathe. Sit IN the energetics of each chakra/energy center for at least 20 minutes. You can do this in silence or, as Venus loves to speak through song lyrics, poetry, sounds, and even lines in movies, it might be that a certain song wants to be played, or a phrase wants to be chanted, or you may want to play a singing bowl. It might be that you have a piece of music that you listen to at

each CHU that activates the remembrance in you that this is your sacred and devotional moon-thly practice.

3. When the 20 minutes are up, use the mirror work practice and heart riff prompts I've offered for each chakra/energetic center. And then I encourage you to witness, feel, and experience what comes up for you and what Self Source-ery is required to support and nourish that exploration.

NOTE: You don't have to do it all. What I share is optional. If astrology isn't your thing, skip that. If you're happy to simply sit in the energy of the CHU each moon-th and receive, brilliant. If you're short on time and/or feel overwhelmed with the idea of… well, all of this, you could just create a mini heart-map ritual at each CHU.

INVITATION:
CREATE A HEART-MAP RITUAL

At each cosmic hook-up, set up your Venus space, light a white candle (or you may want to light a candle that's associated with the chakra color you're working with, or have an item on your altar to represent that color.) Take out your journal and pen and your mirror and give yourself at least 20 minutes to enter IN with what wants to be revealed THROUGH you.

This is literally a create-your-own SHE quest, so please, make it your own!

Morning star Venus/the descent cosmic hook-ups (CHUs)

1st CHU

❋ Chakra: Crown

❋ Color: Violet

❋ Key theme: Authority/agency/sovereignty

Set up your space, get comfy, bring your attention to the body area of this chakra/energy center, and give yourself 20 minutes of stillness to simply breathe and receive. Be. Here. NOW. Follow these set-up instructions for the 2nd to 7th CHUs.

Astrological sign

Make a note of the astrological sign of this CHU. What are the main traits/power points and hotspots associated with it? You can use a search engine or an astrology app to find a brief description of each astrological sign. Now think about those in terms of this chakra/energy center and what it represents. Are they harmonious or do they challenge each other? Follow these instructions for the 2nd to 7th CHUs.

Mirror work practice

To set up, feel yourself grounded, IN your body, and now look at yourself in the mirror. Remember to breathe, stay present, feel, and witness what comes up for you, and let this process be a loving and nourishing one. Let your face soften as you look into your own eyes. Follow these set-up instructions for the 2nd to 7th CHUs.

For the 1st CHU, think of the word 'power.' Repeat it over and over again out loud and witness how that feels in your body and being. Many of us have an interesting relationship with the idea of power, so as you bring your attention to your crown chakra, and if, like Inanna, you surrender your golden crown – which is ultimately your connection to the divine realms – are you *still* able to recognize that YOU are powerful and divine? Does that feel possible? To activate and affirm, place a hand on your heart, keep looking into your own eyes and repeat three times: ***I am powerful, and I am divine.***

Heart riff prompts

You can take the mirror work practice to your journal and share what feels and sensations you experienced as you did it and/or you can riff with your heart on the following questions. (Again, follow these instructions for the heart riff prompts I share in the 2nd to 7th CHUs.)

* What's my current relationship with power and the divine? Are they very separate? Does one support the other?

* What is self-power and what does it FEEL like?

* What are the ways I recognize myself AS divine?

What Self Source-ery do you require?

What are some of the ways that you can tend to, satiate, and support yourself as you explore your relationships with power and the divine?

2nd CHU

* Chakra: Third eye

* Color: Purple

* Key theme: Perception/inner vision

Follow the set-up instructions in the 1st CHU.

Astrological sign

Follow instructions in the 1st CHU.

Mirror work practice

Follow the set-up instructions in the 1st CHU. Bring your attention to your third eye and ask for your inner tuition, your inner vision, to become activated. Feel a warmth start to occur at this space as you let your attention rest there. Now, keeping your head still, let your gaze move to your peripheral vision, the space just that little bit further than you can physically see (to the space where the magic sparks and possibility occurs.)

Now if, like Inanna, you surrender your lapis and pearl forehead chain here – which is ultimately your inner vision, your oracular and sensorial nature – are you *still* able to look at your reflection and remember, and more importantly, trust, that you and your body would, and can, STILL KNOW? Does that feel possible?

To activate and affirm, place a hand on your heart, keep looking into your own eyes and repeat three times: *I trust my body's deep wisdom and gnostic knowing to see in the dark.*

Heart riff prompts

Follow the set-up instructions in the 1st CHU.

❋ Close your eyes and ask your body: Who am I? Not your name or your occupation. Wait, and then write down the first thoughts, feelings, and sensations that come through you. You may surprise yourself.

❋ What does my body KNOW, right now, to be TRUE?

❋ What is at my peripheral vision that wants to be explored?

What Self Source-ery do you require?

What are some of the ways that you can tend to, satiate, and support yourself as you explore your relationships with your intuitive nature and body wisdom and knowing?

3rd CHU

❋ Chakra: Throat

❋ Color: Blue

❋ Key theme: Communication/voice

Follow the set-up instructions in the 1st CHU.

Astrological sign

Follow the instructions in the 1st CHU.

Mirror work practice

Follow the set-up instructions in the 1st CHU. Repeat your name as a mantra, to your reflection. What tone do you speak it in? Is it authoritative? Try singing it – does it feel different? Addressing ourselves, speaking our name as a power mantra, is a way to make our voice and our presence known, both to ourselves and to the world.

Now if, like Inanna, you surrender your lapis necklace here – which ultimately is your voice and expression – are you *still* able to look at your reflection and know that your voice, your story, and the words you speak and express matter? Does that feel possible?

To activate and affirm, place a hand on your heart, keep looking into your own eyes and repeat three times: *I (insert your full name here) and the words that I speak and express matter.*

Heart riff prompts

Follow the set-up instructions in the 1st CHU.

* How do I speak to myself about myself? How does it feel to receive that?

* Is the voice that I speak to myself in my own or does it belong to another – real or imagined? Take a moment to really listen.

* How do I express myself to others? Do I hold back or are they receiving my fullest expression and story?

What Self Source-ery do you require?

What are some of the ways that you can tend to, satiate, and support yourself as you explore your relationships with your voice and being heard?

4th CHU

* Chakra: Heart

* Color: Green

* Key theme: Compassion/love

Follow the set-up instructions in the 1st CHU.

Astrological sign

Follow the instructions in the 1st CHU.

Mirror work practice

Follow the set-up instructions in the 1st CHU. Hold your gaze and place a hand on your heart. Breathe into the space under your palm and feel the sensation of warm, gooey, sensual honey. In the middle is a green emerald and it's pulsating pure mother love. Let the pulse move out from your heart and fill your entire body with pure mother love. If there are stiff and stuck parts, if there are places and spaces of resistance, simply keep sending more there.

Now if, like Inanna, you surrender your breastplate, your emotional heart – which ultimately is your ability to love yourself and love others – are you *still* able to look at your reflection and know that you're both worthy AND capable of love? To activate and affirm, place a hand on your heart, keep looking into your own eyes and repeat three times: *I am both worthy and capable of love.*

Heart riff prompts

Follow the set-up instructions in the 1st CHU.

* How does my heart want me to feel about myself?

* How can I connect more deeply with my heart?

* When I trust my heart as my compass, it wants me to… (close your eyes, wait, and when you open them, write your response without letting your head get in the way.)

What Self Source-ery do you require?

What are some of the ways that you can tend to, satiate, and support yourself as you explore your relationships with your heart, with yourself, and with others?

5th CHU

❋ Chakra: Solar plexus

❋ Color: Yellow

❋ Key theme: Personal power

Follow the set-up instructions in the 1st CHU.

Astrological sign

Follow the instructions in the 1st CHU.

Mirror work practice

Follow set-up instructions in the 1st CHU. Place a hand on your solar plexus. This is a sensitive spot for many of us; I've always held a lot of physical weight here as protection, to keep people at a distance because of previously leaky boundaries. Hold your gaze and allow yourself to sit or stand straighter and taller, feet on the ground, and breathe deeper.

Look at the powerful person staring back at you right now. Remember and recognize yourself as powerful. Remember and recognize yourself as someone who has boundaries. Remember and recognize yourself as someone who always has a choice. Feel how this version of you wants to stand and sit.

Maintain eye contact with your gaze and lift your chin. We've got so used to taking selfies from above because it's 'flattering,' and yet it creates a sense of smallness in our being. Place your mirror in alignment with your solar plexus, lift your chin, and now look down at your reflection. POWERFUL.

Now if, like Inanna, you surrender your golden lasso/hip chain – which is your personal power – are you *still* able to trust and KNOW that you are powerful and have choice and autonomy over your body AND your experience? Does that feel possible? To activate and affirm, place a hand on your heart, keep looking into your own eyes, and repeat three times: *I am powerful, and I always have the power to choose.*

Heart riff prompts
Follow the set-up instructions in the 1st CHU.

* Where do I hold strong boundaries in life and where am I leaky?

* Do I know what I want and how to ask for it? What would THAT look and feel like?

* If I believed that I always have the power to choose, what would I do differently?

What Self Source-ery do you require?
What are some of the ways that you can tend to, satiate, and support yourself as you explore your relationships with your personal power and boundaries?

6th CHU

* Chakra: Sacral

* Color: Orange

* Key theme: Sensuality/creativity

Follow the set-up instructions in the 1st CHU.

Astrological sign

Follow the instructions in the 1st CHU.

Mirror work practice

Follow the set-up instructions in the 1st CHU. Hold your gaze and bring your attention to your sacral space. Physically, it's the place just beneath your belly button, but energetically, it always feels to me like my entire pelvic bowl, my medicine maker, my cauldron of creation. Continue to hold your gaze, while slowly, really slowly, rotating your hips. First in one direction, then in the other. I call this 'stirring the cauldron' and it's a simple yet effective way to move our creative and sensual energy. You're a creative being and it's through what you create – whether that's life itself, projects, art, a home, or a loving environment for others – that you really can recognize the potency of your creative and sensual power.

Now if, like Inanna, you surrender your ankle bracelets – which represent your creativity and value – are you *still* able to trust and KNOW that you're a Creatrix whose creations in the world hold value? Does that feel possible? To activate and affirm, place a hand on your heart, keep looking into your own eyes, and repeat three times: **I am a Creatrix. I value myself and all that I create.**

Heart riff prompts

Follow the set-up instructions in the 1st CHU.

❋ What creations are currently wanting to be brought into manifest through me?

❋ Where do I feel that my values are most challenged?

❋ What are my five most important values in this lifetime? Are they interchangeable or absolutely non-negotiable? What do they say about who I am as a person?

What Self Source-ery do you require?

What are some of the ways that you can tend to, satiate, and support yourself as you explore your relationships with your sensuality and creativity?

7th CHU

❋ Chakra: Root

❋ Color: Red

❋ Key theme: Life force/source

Follow the set-up instructions in the 1st CHU.

Astrological sign

Follow the instructions in the 1st CHU.

Mirror work practice

Follow the set-up instructions in the 1st CHU. Bring your attention to your root, to the power center between your thighs. Place a hand there if you need a reminder of the power that resides there. Hold your gaze and breathe all the way in, through the nose, past the heart, past your belly, right down deep into your root. On the out-breath, let the air release but keep the attention there. Do this five times. You're holding your gaze and rooting into your root with the breath.

Now if, like Inanna, you surrender your royal robe – representing *all* of who you are – are you *still* able to trust and KNOW that you (insert your name here) are here, IN your body, rooted in the truth of ALL that you are, and whole? Does that feel possible? To activate and affirm, place a hand on your heart, keep looking into your own eyes, and repeat three times: ***I (insert your name) am here, IN my body, and I am whole.***

Heart riff prompts
Follow the set-up instructions in the 1st CHU.

* Am I nourished and satiated at my root? How do I/would I know? What would I need to do to know?

* Trees and plants can't exist without a strong root network, and neither can I. What support do I have? What are some of the key things that create a sense of stability and security in my life?

What Self Source-ery do you require?
What are some of the ways that you can tend to, satiate, and support yourself as you explore your relationships with your roots and foundations?

If there's an 8th CHU

* Key theme: Energetics

Follow the set-up instructions in the 1st CHU.

Astrological sign
Follow the instructions in the 1st CHU.

Mirror work practice

Follow the set-up instructions in the 1st CHU. Hold your gaze in the recognition that you're preparing to INTENTIONALLY enter the underworld. It's YOUR choice. Because from crown to root, you know that despite having surrendered all your accessories, you're whole. Yes, you're naked and vulnerable, yet *still* you know that you're here, in your body and wholly complete.

Whatever your relationship with death, this is a metaphorical one – one in which we choose to release all the labels and ideas and stories that have been put on us, leaving only what's real and true. Breathe that in, hold both your gaze and your breath for the count of three, and then release the breath noisily. Do this three times. You're making space for what's to come.

Now if, like Inanna, you intentionally CHOOSE to enter the underworld – which represents a death to all that's no longer you – are you *still* able to trust and KNOW that you (insert your name here) actively choose to accept a death to all that's no longer you in order to experience what it is to be fully alive in ALL of your becoming? To activate and affirm, place a hand on your heart, keep looking into your own eyes, and repeat three times: ***I (insert your name here) die to ALL that no longer serves me so that I can embrace ALL that I'm becoming.***

Heart riff prompts

Follow the set-up instructions in the 1st CHU.

* Where am I still hiding behind armor and numbing myself? (Radical honesty is required here.)

* What is my relationship with death – both real and metaphorical?

✳ Does anything need to be recognized, honored, and fully released before I enter the underworld?

What Self Source-ery do you require?

What are some of the ways that you can tend to, satiate, and support yourself as you explore your relationship with death – real and metaphorical?

NOTE: Be honest and be kind to yourself here. Ma of the Dark Matter WILL hold you and she will expect to be met with the truth, YOUR truth. She doesn't judge, but she does require and expect honesty and real truth.

Final notes on the morning star phase

It's a choice to descend so please keep honoring and giving yourself a wink of recognition every time you say 'yes' to a mirror practice, every time you *choose* to heart riff at a cosmic hook-up. Because these choices strengthen YOUR rhythmic intelligence, your deepest body wisdom and knowing, and create the deepest remembrance of, and trust in, WHO YOU ARE.

Trust who you are underneath the armor, the stories, the labels.

Mother-loving, courageous, big-hearted YOU.

The archetypal morning star

Morning star Venus is the warrior, she's courage, she's Joan of Arc – she's the source-ed force that can and will move us through the disillusionment and doubts of These Times and into a deep trust (and faith) in what it is that we're cocreating here and now.

It's a time to make bold moves and begin our brave descent into the underworld. I say brave because at this point, it IS brave. (When we return as the evening star, after our time in the underworld, I'd suggest we're bold – there's a difference. I invite you to explore that difference as you experience the Venus cycle in her wholeness.)

I refer to Joan of Arc because A, I LOVE a French heroine and B, she's VERY much a Wild Rose. I've been intrigued by her since I went on a school trip to Rouen, the city in France where she was burned at the stake. Yes, we saw the cathedral that Monet painted, and yes, it was nice, but it was really the story of Joan that stayed with me. And most of all, it was her courage and bravery for daring to stand for what she believed in.

At the age of 17 Joan set out on her mission – guided only by celestial voices, direct from source – to reconquer France. She knew NOTHING about war, yet she was able to reunite and re-engage a previously 'broken' French army and lead them to victory against the English. I MEAN!

Now, I'm 'English,' although it's rarely if ever a label I'd accept as my own, but I remember as a 15-year-old girl being told this story by an overenthusiastic French tour guide who was getting glorious delight from it, and our English teacher trying to somehow 'soften' the blow for us. Yet I cared very little about the 'victory' and became super interested in this female soldier who my English teacher deemed a 'witch.'

Yes, I believe Joan *was* a witch, AND she was, and frankly still is, the most famous female soldier in history. She was brave as fuck and followed her connection to, and the voice of, her source power. I LOVE remembering this story. I LOVE how brave I've been this lifetime because I learned at the age of 15 who Joan of Arc was.

I LOVE how passionate the French guide had been – proud, even, of a young woman who dared to rally an army and claim victory over the English. I LOVE how it made me aware of the word 'heresy' and how that word has been a guiding force for me ever since. Because so often, when I've heard a woman speak a truth that didn't comply with the societal narrative – a narrative dictated ultimately by the tenets of religion – she's been accused of heresy and/or witchcraft.

Now, while I was writing this book, Joan called to me and in my dreamtime she said: 'Come get some burning woman medicine' (in my dreams she was made of molten bronze). A ferry to France leaves daily from where my husband and I live, and he suggested we pack the car and drive to Rouen. So, we did. (I LOVE THAT HOT VIKING.)

I THOUGHT I wanted to go to the site where Joan had prayed before battle, which is about 40 minutes outside Paris, mainly because there was a part of me that thought *Why would I go to the place where she, y'know, BURNED?!!* I'm a FEELER and often when I visit sacred sites, I can not only see and witness in my mind's eye what occurred there, I can also FEEL it. But SHE called loud: 'Come to Rouen' and so we stayed right in the city center. It was still just as beautiful as I remembered it from that school trip. Have you been? I really recommend it.

In Rouen, they revere Joan of Arc and all that she stood for – liberation, freedom, and truth – and honor her as THEIR warrior. They've built a church dedicated to her at the site where she was executed, and that's where I was directly called to go as soon as we arrived. It was SO POWERFUL. Although they burned Joan, that heart of hers, it would NOT burn (despite them trying THREE times) and it's still VERY much alive. There's a bronze statue of Joan as you walk toward the church's altar and her stance – defiant and ON PURPOSE – is the one she held in my dream.

I lit a candle for US – for *all* the women who have been called witches, who have been accused of heresy, burned, literally and metaphorically, in this life and past lives. Then, in front of a beauty-full Madonna, I sat in Joan's church journaling for hours on her/my/our burning woman medicine, until my hand was sore. The Madonna holds a baby in one hand and Joan's heart in the other – the heart that represents the heart of us all, the burning women. The heart that WILL NOT BURN (no matter what). It was such a remembrance that, as my love, author Meggan Watterson, always says: love wins. ALWAYS.

We KNOW that the burning simply makes a place and space for MORE of what's real and true because the Great Mumma holds the hearts of all the burning women who trust themselves and honor their hearts.

Phase: underworld Venus

Venus has moved behind the sun and is invisible to us on Earth for around 50ish days. Are you ready to enter IN? As Venus moves, still as the morning star but invisibly behind the sun, we, like Inanna, enter the underworld. IN to the body to seek our wisdom from within.

Because yes, like Inanna, we've surrendered all the associations and identifications we have with the outside world and are left with the realest of real and the truthiest of truth. This is NOT always comfortable. Rarely, if ever, in fact. It's not meant to be. It's scratchy, raw, and exposed. And our 'work' here is to sit with THAT. The discomfort of being raw and exposed to the queen of the underworld, what some call our shadow self but who I call Ma of the Dark Matter. Because for me, it's only in the dark, in the total unknown, that we can really be honest about what it is we DO know and claim it.

As I shared in my book *Self Source-ery*, Ma of the Dark Matter is the initiate force of transformation and in Her presence, all there EVER is to do is surrender. Yes, there's discomfort and you'll find that, if you slow all the way down, there's GOLD in the discomfort - you may not discover it right away, but in the surrender, you allow yourself to at least be open to discovering it.

But you do have to REALLY drop it all. You can't simply pay lip service to the process. Drop the masks, the pretense, the outdated versions of yourself, the thoughts, beliefs, and ideas of who you are, what you think 'should' be happening in the world, all your judgments about how you and other people should be doing things, and how you/they should be showing up; drop all the ranty comments on social media, all the instructions for what you should say, be, or do in order to be a 'good' person. And surrender. Surrender it all.

It can get grief-y here. Really grief-y. And grief can and will dismantle any structure or 'idea' of how we think it 'should' be. But it will also, if you let it, reveal yourself to you. We don't have to pretend that it's not scary or fearful; as I've said, we have so few rituals and ways in our society to support the process of grief and yet, its revealment is a potent and necessary bringer of alchemy and change.

NOTE: As always, I want to be clear that everything I share here is an invitation. If you're experiencing the darkest of dark spaces while reading this, it might be all you can do to get yourself out of bed - if that's the case, look in the mirror, give yourself a wink and a nod of loving recognition for doing *that*, and soothe yourself in a way that feels good for you.

Surrender IN

Like Inanna, we enter the darkness of the underworld, and the invitation is to surrender. In the story, Erishkigal hangs her sister on a meat hook – but the good news is you don't have to do THAT. We can, however, take this time, in the darkness of our own womb, in the void of the cosmic womb, to really know who we are HERE.

So often, we want to rush out of the underworld, the darkness, the discomfort. Yet, when we truly surrender IN to the well of grief (remembering that anywhere there's a well, there's source power) there's an opportunity to dissolve and transform. It's where the unbearable can become bearable. It's alchemical. Don't push, don't force, allow yourself to be in the deep darkness. It's a nourishing process – being in the vulnerable depths of it all.

It's in the dark, the chaotic, and the unknown that I shed. I grow. I root. I thrive.

Can you sit a little longer in the dark, to find out what REALLY wants to live in you? Yes, it's intense AND… intense doesn't necessarily mean BAD. Think of it as like the things you're passionate/care about being amplified, as if the Black Madonna, Ma of the Dark Matter, of Earth and body and the mystery in between, is pulling you close and whispering (or shouting): *Stop playing small. YOU matter. AND… now let go and release ALL that doesn't.*

I won't lie, and this might FEEL like the sticky part: She DOES mean ALL. Because, what I'm realizing, more and more – in particular on my own Wild Rose Venus path, when I get real and truth-y with myself – is that in order to really ride the wild waves of THESE times, we have to bring our attention to matter: our fleshy body. It's our home and we need to love on it, nurture and nourish it, because we REALLY matter and we must align with our heart (the heart which, like Joan of Arc's, won't burn) and ONLY show up to life, to each other, from THAT place. Because that's really ALL that *actually* matters.

And what doesn't matter? It has to go. THAT is what needs to burn. Let ALL that does NOT matter burn to make space for the opportunities and possibilities that previously may have felt TOO big or TOO bold. THEY matter. Because YOU MATTER.

As in the retrograde phase, underworld Venus has three phases: before cazimi (BC); the cazimi (TC); and after cazimi (AC).

Before cazimi (BC)

Use this time as Venus travels behind the sun, becoming invisible, to REALLY get ruthless in your pursuit of truth and love. Yes, there will be resistance, so recognize it AND continue to get ruthless. The truthier you get with yourself in this phase the more mulch you'll have to alchemize into pure gold.

* What STILL wants to be released?

* Where is fear still living and taking up space within you?

* What would you need to know in order to REALLY let it go and surrender to the darkness?

The cazimi (TC)

This is when Venus is furthest from Earth and so our connection to her can also feel distant, even non-existent, at this point. We really are in the dark and we must trust ourselves, our Self Source-ery – as source power – to navigate the dark.

INVITATION:
ENTER THE VOID

If it feels safe to do so, and if you're called, make some time to be in the dark. REALLY in the dark.

- *Sit in a darkened room wearing an eye mask (and with no music playing) and set a timer for between 15 and 30 minutes. Even the idea of doing this might feel a little edgy – you know you, so trust that. If five minutes feels enough, let it be enough. The invitation is to let what still brings you fear meet you here so it can really, truly be released, leaving a void.*

- *Remember that in the void of NO thing, ANYTHING is possible.*

- *Let yourself, in the dark, reconcile with ALL your parts. Give yourself fierce compassion and let a spark of intention be ignited and blessed with the ancestral wisdom of the darkness and the void, ready for the rebirth. You, in the essence of evening star Venus – wise, all-knowing queen. LIVE into those wishes, create their existence through YOU, as full-spectrum, life-living, glorious woman!*

After cazimi (AC)

Venus is preparing to move out from behind the sun; Inanna is preparing to leave the underworld; and anyone who bleeds KNOWS that feeling of shedding in the darkness of the cosmic womb. To move from one phase to another, after shedding, releasing… well, there's trepidation and a deeper wisdom, and it's what we all experience collectively as Venus prepares to emerge from her time in the underworld, initiated as the dark always does, ready to ascend as the evening star.

But let's not rush ahead. The joy of this cycle is that there's no goal or end result: Instead, it's a cyclical ebb and flow that allows for unfolding and revealment. And it's here, in this AC period of Venus in the underworld, before Venus reappears in the evening sky, that we can really plant our dream seeds of potential in the darkness – audaciously hopeful seeds of intention for the rebirth.

Final notes on the underworld phase

When you're IN a phase of darkness in your life (and remember, the initiatory experience that brings each of us IN *will* be different, so please DON'T consider whether your darkness is MORE or LESS dark than someone else's – that's NOT how this works), it WILL feel as if it may never bloody end. But it does. It really does.

You've done this a thousand times before. You've kept score, so that THIS lifetime is the lifetime you don't simply survive; this is the lifetime where you *choose* to thrive. The lifetime where you *choose* to flourish, nourished. (And satiated and FULL. OF. IT.)

Let this phase of the Venus cycle remind you that it is ALWAYS darkest before the dawn, but the dawn DOES come, the light DOES return, and we DO rise, rooted. It's here that we get stretchy, and we're able to ready ourselves for growth into new and expansive places with love. In service to love. ALL THE LOVE.

INVITATION:
SELF SOURCE

In times of transition – and that's what this part of the Venus cycle can REALLY teach us about the most – there are three practices that I use to navigate and to self-support and source myself on my Wild Rose path.

1. Gratitude, blessings, and miracles

When you're in the not-knowing of a situation or experience, when disappointment or fear may be showing up, ask yourself to track all the ways that this moment and situation are blessing you up. This is a muscle that needs to be stretched and keep being stretched regularly. As Wild Rose, writer, and activist Gloria Steinem said, 'The truth will set you free, but first it will piss you off!' Same is true of this situ – when you're in it, those miracles and blessings can feel non-existent, but they WILL be there. Actively seek them out and give fierce love and gratitude to the experience. (FYI: No one's saying don't get pissed off – absolutely feel ALL the feels, and STILL give thanks for the miracles and blessings. It's ALL available here.)

2. Rhythms and rituals

I say this often, but when they took away our rituals, they took away our power. So when we find ways to restore our rhythmic nature, it makes it so much easier to remember our capacity for magic. Especially if we're experiencing a phase of darkness. Returning to and honoring daily habits (keep them super simple) as rhythms and rituals helps us to stay reconnected and IN our bodies, alive and awake to the entire experience of life: the ebb and the flow, the longings and desires, the fullness of the feminine expression. We are then able to prioritize a deeper connection to our personal values and worth: create, dance, sing, support others. Make moves from THAT place.

3. Sound codes are Venus codes

Speak power and magic over yourself when you wake up. Listen to music/ audiobooks by people who inspire you and make you feel supported and nourished. Read and/or write devotional words to yourself, for yourself, before turning your phone on each morning. By actively tuning in to and creating supportive frequencies we're able to intentionally move our energy and thoughts in the direction of love each day.

Phase: evening star Venus/the ascent

Evening star Venus is the return of the queen to her throne. She's the Source-ress of remembered magic who, having surrendered to death, is now ready to fully live and experience it all. As morning star Venus, we were brave, and we dared to take risks. But now, as evening star Venus, we're bold – we Self Source, we're intentional, and we prioritize pleasure, art, beauty, and life-living FULLY.

This phase is the rebirth, renaissance, and reclamation of the revealment of self-trust and self-power that we discovered in the darkness. The truth of who we are and the power that resides there. We develop a confidence and an inner security in our relationship with self and also with those around us. And we're much more likely to choose quality over quantity in terms of… well, everything: from the food we eat to the friends we make, to how we spend our time.

For me, this is where we experience the difference between brave and bold. Brave is descending, feeling the burn, entering IN and meeting Ma of the Dark Matter. Brave is sitting in the void of NO thing, of not-knowing, of uncertainty, and staying with it. So that the emergence, the ascent, is rooted. Because it's in the darkness that we grow our strongest roots – there's a trust in ourselves, what we've experienced, what it is we know, and it's here that we get bold. SO, while I feel that Wild Rose Joan of Arc is very much the archetypal morning star, it's the emboldened Wild Rose Mary Magdalene who is evening star.

It's in this phase that we get to realize and recognize the Magdalene IN each of us. **IN OUR BODIES. IN OUR EXPERIENCES.**

The times we've been blamed. Shamed. Silenced. Shh-ed. Censored. Cancelled. Not believed. Sexualized. Devalued. Not trusted. Been made to feel worthless and unlovable. Been told that we *need* to be 'redeemed.' I know YOU can add a trillion more variations on this. All the ways in which your/our love and magic and power have been deemed TOO dangerous and TOO powerful in attempts (in MANY cases, really bloody successful ones) to make you/us no longer trust and/or believe ourselves. Or each other.

They've disconnected us from our bodies, from our rhythmic and cyclical intelligence; they've told us that we need outside sources to access divinity so that we no longer trust or believe in the love, magic, and power that resides IN OUR BODIES.

I've spoken about this in many ways in EVERY book I've written, but Mary Magdalene returns us to the heart of the matter, THE HEART OF MATTER. YOUR body AS matter, because YOU matter – making all of the connections between her and Cassandra and Cleopatra and Hathor and Isis and Madonna. It's ALL CONNECTED. It's ALL MAGDALENE. And it's as the evening star that the BOLD act of self-power reclamation REALLY happens.

Evening star Venus CHU steps

1. As Venus makes her monthly cosmic hook-ups with the now waxing (growing bigger) crescent moon, we too ascend, and on the way, we're honoring, reclaiming, and revering our potency and power at each gate. As it did on the descent, each CHU will occur in a different astrological sign. Refer to your chosen astrological app for a daily forecast. Again, each CHU will occur in the same chakra/energetic center order, ascending from bottom to top, root to crown, through the seven chakra/energy centers. At each one I invite you to create a ritual/time-out-of-time to connect IN with this experience.

2. Locate the chakra/energy center on your body – place a hand there if it helps – bring your attention to that area and breathe. Sit IN the energetics of each chakra/energy center for at least 20 minutes. As before, you can do this in silence or play a song or a singing bowl; or it might be that you listen to a particular piece of music at each CHU that activates the remembrance in you that this is your sacred and devotional moon-thly practice.

3. When those 20 minutes are up, use the mirror work practice and heart riff prompts I share for each chakra/energetic center. And then witness, feel, and experience what comes up for you and what Self Source-ery is required to support and nourish that exploration. Working with the rhythmic intelligence of Venus, creating your own Self Source-ery through ritual and ceremony, supports you to come into harmony with that.

NOTE: Again, if you're short on time and/or overwhelmed with the idea of all of this, you can create a mini heart-map ritual at each CHU as Venus ascends; *see page 141.*

Evening star Venus/the ascent cosmic hook-ups (CHUs)

7th CHU

❋ Chakra: Root

❋ Color: Red

❋ Key theme: Life force/source

Set up your space, get comfy, bring your attention to the body area of this energy center and give yourself 20 minutes of stillness to simply breathe and receive. Be. Here. NOW. Follow these set-up instructions for the 6th to 1st CHUs.

Astrological sign

Make a note of the astrological sign of this CHU. What are the main traits/power points and hotspots associated with it? Now think about those in terms of this chakra/energy center and what it represents. Are they harmonious or do they challenge each other? Follow these instructions for the 6th to 1st CHUs.

Mirror work practice

To set up, feel yourself grounded, IN your body, and now look at yourself in the mirror. Remember to breathe, stay present, feel, and witness what comes up for you and to let this process be a loving and nourishing one. Let your face soften as you look into your own eyes. Follow these set-up instructions for the 6th to 1st CHUs.

Bring your attention to your root, to the power center between your thighs. Place a hand there if you need a reminder of the power that resides there. Hold your gaze and breathe all the way in, through the nose, past the heart, past your belly, right down deep into your root. On the out-breath, let the air release, but keep the attention there. Do this five times. You're holding your gaze and rooting into your root with the breath.

Now if, like Inanna, you reclaim your royal robe – which represents all of who you are – are you *still* able to trust and KNOW that either with OR without it, you (insert your name here) are here, IN your body, rooted in the truth of ALL that you are? And that you're ALL of your parts – the so-called light AND dark – and that you're whole? You'd better bloody believe it! To activate and affirm, place a hand on your heart, keep looking into your own eyes, and repeat three times: *I (insert your name here) own and reclaim all my parts – I'm whole.*

Heart riff prompts

You can take the mirror practice to your journal and share what feels and sensations you experienced as you did the practice and/or you can riff with your heart on the following questions. Follow these instructions for the heart riff prompts in the 6th to 1st CHUs.

* How can I prioritize MY own needs, wants, and desires (so that I CAN be a strong container and support for others)?

* Can I place LOVE at MY own foundations – what would that look and feel like?

* What are my non-negotiables when deepening my relationship with stability – physically and emotionally?

What Self Source-ery do you require?

What are some of the ways that you can tend to, satiate, and support yourself as you reclaim, strengthen, and deepen your relationships with your roots and foundations?

6th CHU

❋ Chakra: Sacral

❋ Color: Orange

❋ Key theme: Sensuality/creativity

Follow the set-up instructions in the 7th CHU.

Astrological sign

Follow the instructions in the 7th CHU.

Mirror work practice

Follow the set-up instructions in the 7th CHU. Hold your gaze and bring your attention to your sacral space. This energy center is situated between your hips and as you hold your own gaze, move your hips, your entire medicine bowl, in a ceremony of reclamation.

Stir your creative life force and dance in remembrance of who you are. You're so mother-loving worthy. You're a Creatrix, SHE who can bring entire universes into being. Hold your gaze and witness yourself as the Creatrix of your own reality, on your terms, in total delicious alignment with your values and beliefs.

Now if, like Inanna, you reclaim your ankle bracelets – which represent your creativity and value – are you *still* able to trust and KNOW that either with OR without them, you're a Creatrix whose creations in the world hold fierce value? You'd better bloody believe it! To activate and affirm, place a hand on your heart, keep looking into your own eyes, and repeat three times: *I create my own reality. I know my worth.*

Heart riff prompts

Follow the set-up instructions in the 7th CHU. Revisit the list of your five most important values that you created in the heart riff prompt in the 6th CHU on the descent; *see page 151*.

❋ Does this list of values still ring true? Or does it need tweaking and amending to account for new developments that occurred in the underworld? Our values are often non-negotiable, but the point of the Venus cycle is to work *with* it in order to create a harmonization in your body and experience. So, don't be afraid to make changes and course correct when and where they're needed.

❋ As the Creatrix of *your* reality, if you're not doing so already, dream into how life could be even more juicy and alive for you. What needs to happen? Get specific.

What Self Source-ery do you require?

What are some of the ways that you can tend to, satiate, and support yourself as you reclaim, strengthen, and deepen your relationships with your values and creativity?

5th CHU

❋ Chakra: Solar plexus

❋ Color: Yellow

❋ Key theme: Personal power

Follow the set-up instructions in the 7th CHU.

Astrological sign

Follow the set-up instructions in the 7th CHU.

Mirror work practice

Follow the set-up instructions in the 7th CHU. Place a hand on your solar plexus, hold your gaze and lift your chin. It's a posture of defiance and knowing. Breathe into it and smile.

Personal power isn't at war with anyone – it's a peace, it's knowing who you are in defiance of all you've been told that you could and should be. Give your defiant knowing a head nod of recognition and maybe even a cheeky wink. Peaceful, potent, delicious self-power? It looks GOOD on you.

Now if, like Inanna, you reclaim your golden lasso/hip chain – your personal power – are you *still* able to trust and KNOW that either with OR without it, you're powerful, and you have choice and autonomy over your body AND your experience? You'd better bloody believe it! To activate and affirm, place a hand on your heart, keep looking into your own eyes, and repeat three times: ***I am defiantly who I choose to be. Me, unapologetically.***

Heart riff prompts

Follow the set-up instructions in the 7th CHU.

❋ Without apology, who AM I? Make this your statement of declaration and turn it into a screen saver on your phone, or a piece of art for your wall. OWN IT!

❋ Defiance is in the knowing. What is it that I KNOW to be true about MY power?

❋ What am I choosing?

What Self Source-ery do you require?

What are some of the ways that you can tend to, satiate, and support yourself as you reclaim, strengthen, and deepen your relationships with your personal power and boundaries?

4th CHU

❋   Chakra: Heart

❋   Color: Green

❋   Key theme: Compassion/love

Follow the set-up instructions in the 7th CHU.

Astrological sign

Follow the set-up instructions in the 7th CHU.

Mirror work practice

Follow the set-up instructions in the 7th CHU. Hold your gaze and place a hand on your heart. Feel the pulse, the ancient rhythm of your entire lineage, of the ancestors of ancient-future, all residing right there at your heart space – supporting, loving, and holding you as you courageously follow your heart, no matter what. Like Mary Magdalene, whose path was one of the deepest, most compassionate love; like me, who has a tattoo of a compass and its true north that points directly to my heart, you too trust your heart as your compass.

Now if, like Inanna, you reclaim your breastplate, your emotional heart – your ability to love yourself and love others – are you *still* able to trust and KNOW that either with OR without it, you're both worthy of AND capable of love? You'd better bloody believe it, beauty-full! To activate and affirm, place a hand on your heart, keep looking into your own eyes, and repeat three times: **My heart is my true north and I follow it always.**

Heart riff prompts

Follow the set-up instructions in the 7th CHU.

* What does my heart want to experience the most?

* Can I listen deeply enough to the yearning of my heart and see what wants to be uncovered? (It's usually found underneath what it is we THINK we want.)

* How do I give my heart what it wants?

What Self Source-ery do you require?

What are some of the ways that you can tend to, satiate, and support yourself as you reclaim, strengthen, and deepen your relationships with your heart, with yourself, and with others?

3rd CHU

* Chakra: Throat

* Color: Blue

* Key theme: Communication/voice

Follow the set-up instructions in the 7th CHU.

Astrological sign

Follow the instructions in the 7th CHU.

Mirror work practice

Follow the set-up instructions in the 7th CHU. Hold your gaze, place a hand lightly on your neck/throat area, and repeat your full name as a power mantra directly to your reflection in your most loving and powerful tone. Feel the vibration of the tone underneath the palm of your hand. Let that vibration move through your entire body.

Your name IS a power mantra that's meant to be spoken. Looking at your reflection and speaking you name as truth and power, letting it vibrate, is both tonal medicine AND a declaration: *I'm here and I'm taking up space and my voice and expression will be heard and experienced.* It's SO BLOODY POWERFUL.

Now if, like Inanna, you reclaim your lapis necklace – your voice and expression – are you *still* able to trust and KNOW that either with OR without it, your voice, your story, and the words you speak and express, matter? You'd better bloody believe it, beauty-full! To activate and affirm, place a hand on your heart, keep looking into your own eyes, and repeat three times: *I am (insert your full name here) and the words I speak are a spell of truth and power.*

Heart riff prompts

Follow the set-up instructions in the 7th CHU.

* What IS my truth?

* If the words I speak are a spell of truth and power, what spell am I currently wanting to weave?

* What would my FULLEST expression sound like? What would its tone be? What language would it use? Would it sing, rap, recite lyrical poetry?

What Self Source-ery do you require?

What are some of the ways that you can tend to, satiate, and support yourself as you reclaim, strengthen, and deepen your relationships with your voice and being heard?

2nd CHU

* Chakra: Third eye
* Color: Purple
* Key theme: Perception/inner vision

Follow the set-up instructions in the 7th CHU.

Astrological sign

Follow the instructions in the 7th CHU.

Mirror work practice

Follow the set-up instructions in the 7th CHU. Maintain your gaze and bring your attention to the space just above and between your eyebrows. Momentarily take your gaze there, hold for a count of three, and then relax your eyes back to meet your gaze in your reflection. You're an oracle. A seer. Like your ancient-future ancestors, you're able to use all of your senses – known and unknown – to 'see' across space and time.

Now if, like Inanna, you reclaim your lapis and pearl forehead chain here – your inner vision, your oracular and sensorial nature – are you *still* able to trust and KNOW that either with OR without it, you and your body would, and can, STILL KNOW? You'd better believe it, beauty-full! To activate and affirm, place a hand on your heart, keep looking into your own eyes, and repeat three times: ***I am an oracle. I see what I know, and I trust what I see.***

Heart riff prompts

Follow the set-up instructions in the 7th CHU.

* What are your inner visions reflecting and projecting?

* Close your eyes and allow your third eye to open fully – what wants to be seen and experienced?

* What is your felt sense of what it is you can 'see'?

What Self Source-ery do you require?

What are some of the ways that you can tend to, satiate, and support yourself as you reclaim, strengthen, and deepen your relationships with your intuitive nature and knowing?

1st CHU

* Chakra: Crown

* Color: Violet

* Key theme: Authority/agency/sovereignty

Follow the set-up instructions in the 7th CHU.

Astrological sign

Follow the instructions in the 7th CHU.

Mirror work practice

Follow the set-up instructions in the 7th CHU. Hold your gaze and recognize that the eyes looking back at you are the eyes of an all-seeing, all-knowing, sourced, satiated, and powerful queen. Now breathe in. Fill your entire body with violet light as you do.

Hold your breath and hold your gaze. Smile at your reflection as you release the breath. Do this three times.

If, like Inanna, you reclaim your golden crown – which is ultimately your connection to the divine realms – are you *still* able to trust and KNOW that either with OR without it, YOU are both powerful and divine? You'd better bloody believe it, beauty-full! To activate and affirm, place a hand on your heart, keep looking into your own eyes, and repeat three times: *I am an all-seeing, all-knowing, sourced, satiated, and powerful queen.*

Heart riff prompts
Follow the set-up instructions in the 7th CHU.

* How can I align and harmonize my divine experience *and* the human lived experience?

* Where is my power needing to be reclaimed, so I remember and KNOW that I am SHE and SHE is me?

* How can I honor and revere MY sovereignty?

What Self Source-ery do you require?
What are some of the ways that you can tend to, satiate, and support yourself as you reclaim, strengthen, and deepen your relationships with power and the divine?

If there's an 8th CHU

* Key theme: Energetics

Follow the set-up instructions in the 7th CHU.

Astrological sign

Follow the instructions in the 7th CHU.

Mirror work practice

Follow the set-up instructions in the 7th CHU. Hold your gaze in the recognition that you're about to move back into the retrograde period, when Venus enters the heart of the sun, preparing to move from evening star back to morning star and begin an entirely new cycle. This is an invitation for you to INTENTIONALLY self-initiate AT your heart. Breathe that in, hold both your gaze and your breath for the count of three, releasing the breath noisily. Do this three times. You're making space for what's to come.

Now if, like Inanna, you're intentionally self-initiating, if you're entering a state of metamorphosis where alchemic change can and will occur, where once again you're actively choosing to be fully alive with all that being fully alive entails – the pain, the beauty, the art, the pleasure, the disillusion, the sadness, the heartbreak and the gazillion other experiences that WILL occur if you choose life – do you still want to… well, choose life? To live WITH the heart intention to live your fullest expression of the wildest of roses? You'd better bloody believe it, beauty-full!

To activate and affirm, place a hand on your heart, keep looking into your own eyes, and repeat three times: *I (insert your name here) choose, with the biggest heart intention, to live the fullest expression of the wildest of roses.*

Heart riff prompts

Follow the set-up instructions in the 7th CHU.

✱ How would life be if you and those connected to you recognized, honored, and revered your gifts, talents, and magic in the world? How would you walk into a room? What would you be wearing?

When I was young, my best friend and I used to pretend we were wearing crowns when we walked into town; we literally walked tall with our heads held high as if we had the heaviest and bling-y-est crowns on. And you DO walk differently. You hold yourself differently and your posture makes you create BQE – Big Queen Energy. Try it.

✱ What would you say? How would people talk to you?

For the longest time, I'd let people cut me off mid-sentence because I've always struggled with speaking out loud. So, when I DO talk, I can often take a little longer to say the thing I want to say. But NO ONE gets to cut you off when you speak, OK? Now if someone tries to do that, I'll either stop speaking and then continue where I was when they finish, OR I'll get cross and make it known that I don't appreciate being cut off mid-sentence.

This part of the Venus cycle – at the meeting point of our auric field, our energetics, our vibration, our frequency – is a cosmic cue that it's OUR time to align and emanate and radiate our divine SHE power.

What Self Source-ery do you require?

What are some of the ways that you can tend to, satiate, and support yourself as you reclaim, strengthen, and deepen your relationships with ALL OF LIFE?

Final notes on the evening star phase

As you come to the end of the evening star experience and re-enter the retrograde phase, please recognize it as a power moment of this Venusian heart-led journey of total mother-loving courage you've been on. You've claimed your throne and your sovereignty and now you're emanating and radiating *all* that you are, with your heart as your compass, ready to navigate an entirely new cycle, with its new set of astrological themes and revealments.

Except, you've now created a living mistress-ry map of YOUR Wild Rose path – the mysteries of YOUR mistress-ry have begun to reveal themselves to you through the cyclical and rhythmic intelligence of Venus. You've taken your throne and crowned yourself queen – because self-initiation is really the only initiation that I get behind – and now it's time to be in service to love: to serve yourself, to serve magic, to serve the mother-loving world.

AND SO IT MOTHER-LOVING IS.

INVITATION:
BREATHE THE VENUS CYCLE

To feel the cycle IN YOUR BODY, I invite you to experience it through the breath. First, get comfy and allow your body to relax and soften. If you have frankincense essential oil, you can use it in a diffuser, or if you know that your skin won't react to it, you can use it to anoint your crown, third eye, throat, heart, and sacral space (below the belly button).

1. Take a look around you and feel and sense your surroundings. If it feels good and safe to do so, close your eyes and bring your attention to your breath. Place a hand on your heart and set the intention to receive the wisdom and codes of the Venus cycle in your body: ***I honor my body as a vessel of love.***

2. Take a deep breath in through the nose for a slow count of five. Come in, come down, past your heart and into the depths of your medicine bowl – hold for a count of three in the darkness and void of No thing and release the breath, up and out through the body and through your mouth for a count of five.

3. The inhale is the descent in and down, the warrior Joan of Arc. The pause in the No thing is the space between, a meeting of Ma of the Dark Matter. The exhale is the rise, FROM the darkness, the queen, Mary Magdalene.

4. Set aside 15 minutes to be WITH this breath, to connect to what's underneath it all, let go, and let something MORE move through you. This is flow state. This is YOU, as Venus. Working deeply with source and matter to support and deeply harmonize with life itself.

The harmonics of the Divine Feminine

I love sharing the Venus cycle mostly because it's available to be felt and experienced through our body. It's a template for *how* to self-initiate (and believe me, it takes a few deaths and rebirths to meet, recognize, and reveal who you *really* are.) To trust in the experiential wisdom of what *you've* lived and felt, because it's that which changes and shapes you. (And it's also HOW you become more discerning – you witness and recognize the difference between those who speak from memorized information and those who share from lived and felt experience: Personally, the latter are the *only* ones I want to be in conversation with!)

To lean into the wholeness of who you are. ALL OF THE PARTS, light and dark and the technicolor experience of existence that lies between - not the person you wish you could be or have been told you should be. You're here for the *whole* of life. Not just the easy or straightforward parts. ALL. OF. IT. The laughter, the tears, the love, the heartbreak, the rain, the sunshine, the magic, the beauty. ALL. OF. IT. It's why I believe that the Venus cycle is the most incredible map to support you on your own sacred path. To refine and define your feminine frequency and to have a sensual love affair with all of life.

Follow your Wild Rose petaled path

Your body is a Venus Mystery School

Your Venus SHE quest will unfurl more of your Venus keys and codes — Venusian mysteries that are medicine and magic being remembered THROUGH you.

Self-initiation

Don't wait for someone to give you permission and/or initiate you. The Venus cycle is self-initiatory, so take your throne and crown yourself a Venusian queen.

Your heart as your compass

While I very much recommend working with the Venus cycle in *all* the ways that I've outlined in this salon, when it comes to *knowing* what's real and true for you, trusting your heart as your compass IS ENOUGH.

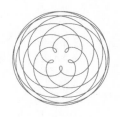

I hold the keys and codes for both death and rebirth, and I'm perpetually becoming – unfolding and unfurling, one Wild Rose petal at a time.

6

WILD ROSE SHE SALON

Dreamscaping and Magic-Making with Venus

'I postpone death by living. By suffering, by
error. By risking. By giving. By loving.'
ANAÏS NIN – FRENCH-AMERICAN AUTHOR

This SHE salon is about remembering our capacity to dream, vision, create, and magic-make for these wild and shifting times. Venus, as a feminine frequency of love and creation, lived and experienced through each of us, is *how* we find, create, and cultivate meaning and purpose, source power and wisdom, intuitive knowing and inspiration – the significance of… well, all of life. Yep, it's *in* the feminine frequency that we find our reason for living.

Born in Paris (of COURSE she was) Anaïs Nin is/was one of THE wildest Roses. She's often referred to as one of *the* finest writers of female erotica, and rightly so. Her book *Delta of Venus*, written in the 1940s and published posthumously in 1977, was groundbreaking in that in it, she dared to create her own 'language of the senses.' Yum.

Anaïs FULLY LIVED and then she wrote it all down. She didn't let others decide who she was, and she didn't have others speak her story *to* her. Her diaries are the most read and reread books on my bookshelves because she speaks to the female experience. In fact, in a postscript to her diary entries, she explains how her desire was to use 'women's language, seeing sexual experience from a woman's point of view.'

A woman seeing, feeling, and expressing herself from HER perspective, in HER own language, about HER own experience should *not* be 'divisive,' 'radical,' or 'controversial,' and yet these are just *some* of the terms that critics have used to describe both Anaïs and her work. Personally, I actively go out of my way to seek out women and humans who are considered to be all of these things; they often turn out to be my favorite people. *Wink.*

Be the Creatrix of your reality

Anaïs Nin was also accused of 'creating her own reality' – as if that was somehow a bad thing. In fact, I feel – and Venus is ALL about the feels – that THIS is our loudest siren call of all. Venus has woven it through time and space, and the Women of the Wild Rose ALL have this in common; in fact, I often wear a necklace, gifted to me by my mumma-in-love, inscribed with the words of Wild Rose and artist Frida Kahlo: 'I paint my own reality.'

AND… it's why Venus, her path, her cycle, and the mysteries within it have been hidden from so many of us. If we don't remember and recognize, reclaim and revere our capacity to dream and vision and create our reality, which is the core of our power and our magic and our innate feminine wisdom – the Venus frequency – we let other people tell us who we are, write our story, and control the narrative. And loves, that is NOT OK.

YOUR reality is the one dreamed, created, painted, and narrated by YOU.

Now, the societal programming can be so strong that we simply can't think beyond our current experience. We're so IN the version of what we're being told and sold is our reality that remembering our magic, our vision, our ability to create and reshape reality can feel impossible. AND yet, we HAVE to. It's *why* we're here.

Look, you don't need me to tell you that These Times are definitely some of the wildest ever. Living in this world can feel like both a horror show AND the most glorious and delicious adventure, and I believe the Venus cycle enables us to witness, in Venus's mirror, our ability and capacity to be with, hold, and respond to both. At the same time. (As well as entertain the entire spectrum of experience that sits between these two polarities.)

To dream. All of the things we've been told are impossible (*especially* those things). To call in and call up all the possibilities that haven't even been dared to be imagined. To see and to vision, and for our bodies to become strong, rooted, satiated, nourished, and Self Source-ed Venus Vessels that can hold and contain AND strengthen and magnetize our magic and power. To gain mistress-ry of ourselves, our bodies, our capacity, our magic and power, and to embody it in service to love.

Dreaming big, calling back my power, and manifesting has NEVER been a problem for me. But holding it – so that it could become sustainable, maintainable, and useful; so that it could potentize in energy, strength, and power – well, *that* most definitely *has* been a problem in the past. In fact, I'm sure this has happened to many of us. We've asked for an incredible work opportunity, more money, or a romantic partner, and we have the capacity to call it up and to call it in. However, ultimately, we may have self-sabotaged that opportunity because we simply didn't have the capacity to hold it. To contain and potentize it.

This is the stuff that can/will drive you to think that you're mad, crazy, and not worthy. It can/will also cause pain and discomfort in your body because when we remember, when we call back our power and our magic from all the places throughout time and space where it's been taken from us and/or we've given it away (knowingly or unknowingly) – and when it DOES return, which it WILL because we're powerful women, witches, and humans – it NEEDS a strong and fecund container to return to.

Choose YOUR Venus story

The Venus cycle became a container for me to explore this and I realized that my own body had to be fully loved on, nourished, and deemed worthy, by me, before I was able to start containing and potentizing my power and magic and living my life in the frequency of Venus, of love and creation. I've always been a magnet for magic, and yet I'd still put off so much of what filled me up, what made my heart big, because I was letting the expectations and projections of others narrate my story. I was doing what I thought I needed to do in order to stay 'safe.'

After I collapsed in Paris, I took this to Ma of the Dark Matter, and it was in the darkness of my own healing process – we always remember/rediscover our best magic when we're in the dark – that She and I let a light shine on the story that wanted to be told: MY Venus story. As I visioned, I saw all that wanted to be loved, created, romanced, and savored – the reality that wanted to be created by me and through me – and it was delicious. SO DELICIOUS.

The ideas, projects, places to visit, my life that was waiting to be fully lived. MY Venus story. It became clear that magic and miracles become MUCH more present and available when you're aligned with what the poet and Wild Rose Mary Oliver calls 'your one precious life.' Ma of the Dark Matter, witnessing my vision, whispered in my ear: *All you have to do is choose.* Yep, *all* – ahem – I had to do was CHOOSE.

I had to CHOOSE to take fierce self-responsibility for all the places and spaces in my life where I was currently NOT in alignment with MY Venus story.

I had to CHOOSE to do it all with the fiercest of love and self-compassion – which meant NO cynical side-eye, finger-pointing, or negative self-talk.

I had to CHOOSE to become intentional about the way that I was going to feel and experience life.

Every day, I now CHOOSE to align and keep aligning with my heart. I CHOOSE to declare myself so bloody worthy of living, breathing, and FULLY experiencing MY Venus story. I CHOOSE to Self Source, nourish, restore, and tend to myself so that my body and my nervous system are able to hold and contain MY Venus story (and to ensure that there's always enough space for the magic and miracles that I've not yet dared to even dream).

I CHOOSE, through the actions I take and the moves that I make, to continually refine and define this entire experience. To follow the cosmic winks and synchronicities. To be curious AND intentional, and to create and narrate my reality in the frequency of Venus, of love.

The Venus devotionals

What helps and supports me to stay intentional and keep aligning with MY Venus story? Venus devotionals – practices and rituals in devotion to me, in the frequency and vibration of love, which, when cultivated, intentionally support the creation and narration of MY Venus story as MY reality. YOUR Venus devotionals will differ from mine because our Venus stories are different. AND there are *some* devotionals – NOURISH, DREAM, VISION, CREATE – that ALL Wild Roses who are dedicated and devoted to creating What Comes Next (that's you/me/US) – absolutely, positively NEED and require.

NOURISH

When I chose to align with the Venus frequency, what became very apparent to me very quickly is that what had previously worked for me, what had felt tried and tested and known, was no longer enough. In order for MORE of you – your magic, creativity, power, and wisdom – to become available, and more importantly, in order for you to sustain it for longer and expand it, prioritizing and amplifying self-care and nourishment of your body, mind, and spirit is non-negotiable.

You ARE worthy

It's been scientifically proven that negative self-talk weakens our physical body. This is NOT COOL – and it's why in the Venus SHE quest, I prioritize the mirror work and activating affirmations. Yes, these may feel basic to those who have been exploring the fields of healing and knowing-yourself-better for some time, but that's because they WORK.

We need to reprogram, Venus style, which means ideally, every day, you'd be writing 12-page love sonnets in devotion to yourself, listing and loving on every single thing that makes you glorious, hot, delicious, and so bloody worthy. Actually, I really DO recommend you do this, at least once, and then turn it into art that you look at, recite, feel, and believe every day. AND in the meantime, repeat after me: *I am glorious. I am hot. I am delicious. I am so bloody worthy.*

Move the way love moves

Look, you don't need me to tell you that moving your body is necessary, but you *might* need me to remind you to do it in ways that feel really fun, delicious, and nourishing. For me, that's dancing my arse off to my three favorite songs EVERY morning or doing an online Bachata class. To you, that might look like hiking or sweating it out at the gym. The emphasis is on whatever feels GOOD. This isn't punishment, its nourishment. OK?

Also, don't be surprised if you find yourself wanting to eat differently. This has been a LONG journey for me but trusting that my body KNOWS what she wants to eat, over what I've been told is 'good' for me, with regard to certain health situations, has definitely taken practice. I've had to build a relationship of trust with my body through Self Source-ery, and it's been revolutionary.

Ultimately, it's tending to our body's needs with compassion. We're not trying to fix, mend, or perfect anything. Instead, we're moving toward vitality, and what the medieval mystic, artist, herbalist, and one of my favorite Wild Roses, Hildegard von Bingen, called 'viriditas' or greenness – the divine creative force that runs through all living things – by prioritizing our pleasure, valuing our health, and continually moving the way love wants us to move. Sigh.

Rooted, real, and true

Stay as close as possible to what's real and rooted and true to you. What I mean by that is, when you *know* what's real and true about you, when you know what you value, what matters to you, keep aligning with THAT. Speak from THAT place. Act and create from THAT place. Everything from the food you eat to the people that you surround yourself with, and from the books you read to the conversations you have, continually ask yourself the question: **Is this rooted, real, and true to me?**

If it's not, course correct. Keep aligning, refining, and defining, and be grateful for the contrasting experiences of life. Because it's these moments of 'Oh no, this is NOT COOL with me' or 'I used to love this, but now I can't stand it' that help to make you aware of what it is that you DO want, need, and desire.

DREAM

Being strong Venus Vessels mean that we can fully absorb the big ideas and possibilities that we dream and that we have the viriditas to birth them into being.

Yep, it's down to us, the Wild Roses, to dream.

Big, wild dreams in the frequency of Venus.

The dreams that you have, for what your life, your community, and this world are *supposed* to be like.

Loves, make those dreams SO BLOODY BIG. MAKE THEM UNREASONABLE, even. (They don't have to make sense; in fact, it's better if they don't.)

Then, with all the love in your heart – and your magic, power, and innate feminine wisdom – dream them into being. Birth What Comes Next.

I first remembered this deeply feminine magic (I'm sure Carl Jung would have totally taken credit for it, but I can pretty much guarantee that the wise women were doing this WAAAAAAAAY before him) when I met what I call the Maltese Dreamer. Since my first encounter with her, I've become what some call a 'conscious dreamer.'

Known as the 'Sleeping Lady,' this almost intact statue of a beautiful, glorious, topless, and ample-hipped Ma woman, lying on her side on a low couch, one enormous right forearm beneath her head, the other draped across her heavy breast, was found in the enormous prehistoric underground sanctuary in Malta known as the Hypogeum.

The ceremonial center of the island, the Hypogeum, a catacomb-like structure, covers around 500 square meters (5,380 feet) across three levels and served as a temple, tomb, and healing place. The main hall led into an oracle room where the temple priestesses/oracles/seers would lie down, set intentions, enter Yoga Nidra/dream states and dream all of life into being.

I visited the Sleeping Lady/Maltese Dreamer statue at the National Museum of Archaeology in Malta's capital, Valletta, and when I bought a replica of her on the way out, the shop assistant wrapped her with such love and told me in hushed, conspiratorial tones, 'She's dreaming to remember.'

Ever since, the Maltese Dreamer has been my icon and my avatar for creating my own dream incubators - intentional imaginal spaces. In my own Traveller lineage, we call this a *Butsi* - a creative visualization process through dreamtime. And in fact, it was/is part of many cultures, including those in ancient Mesopotamia, Egypt, Greece, and Australia, and is done both solo and in community to weave our collective dreams and visions into reality.

Tea and dreaming

I held very intentional solo dream incubators for this book at each cosmic hook-up. I began by brewing a cup of Venusian herbs - rose and blue lotus flower - and then I created a gorgeous nest space with cushions and blankets. Next, I burned dream-inducing frankincense incense, dimmed the lights, and anointed my third eye, throat, heart, solar plexus, and navel with rose oil.

I set a clear intention for the dreamscape in my journal, intentionally sipped my tea, and when I was ready, I slipped on a silky eye mask - à la Wild Rose Holly Golightly in the movie *Breakfast at Tiffany's* - and got comfy. This IS a Venusian practice, after all. Sometimes I'd make a dreamscape playlist, while other times, I'd listen to my own drum and sistrum recording as I entered a contained imaginal dream space for between 20 and 50 minutes. And when it was complete, I'd allow space to write directly from source, as source.

NOTE: Blue lotus is an Egyptian herb - the herb of the Creatrix Ma goddess Hathor, herself - which I believe is having a renaissance to support us as we ALL remember and reclaim through OUR Venus frequency.

Sadly, we can't all gather on that delicious Ma island of Malta together under the moon and Venus and collectively dream our Venus stories together. But we ARE connected, through this book, through our Wild Rose paths, through Venus and her cycles, and we can set the intention at each Venus–moon cosmic hook-up, or every time Venus enters a new astrological sign, to be open to receive, through our dreamtime; to begin our own Venusian dream weaving.

INVITATION:
CREATE A VENUSIAN DREAM INCUBATOR

There's nothing to DO here except be open to receive. We're looking to find the threads that are woven through us in dreamtime, so that we create our own divinely woven dream tapestry that will support us ALL.

1. *Before you go to bed make sure you have pen and paper/a journal close by and write the date on a clean page. If you're called, you can make a note of which astrological signs the moon and Venus are in too.*

   I do this so that I can start to map and track patterns and themes and their elemental qualities based on the astrological sign in which they are dreamed. So, for example, if the moon and Venus are in Sagittarius during a morning star Venus phase, Sagittarius is a Fire sign, and morning star Venus is about being brave and introspection, so I make a note that whatever comes through in dreamtime may want to ignite an idea or burn up an old belief. If you menstruate, you may want to mark where you are in your cycle too, as that can offer up very specific-to-you intel about YOUR Venus story.

2.   *Now write the following statement, three times: Tonight, my dream will hold magic and medicine for me AND for the Collective. Let me remember it.*

3.   *When you wake in the morning, note down ANYTHING you remember from your dreams – colors, words, scenarios, symbols, places, timelines. It doesn't have to make sense. In fact, it rarely does. Just write as quickly as you can before it runs through your fingers like sand and/or your conscious mind gets in the way.*

4.   *Start to collect your dreams for an entire Venus cycle and get curious about what story is being woven through you. If you're called, come join us in the SHE Power Collective, where we share our dreams for the COLLECTIVE WEAVE, together.*

VISION

When we declare ourselves a dream weaver, we set in motion a remembering that's woven through time and space, through lineage and legacy, and it's how our ability to 'see' and to then consciously vision is activated.

All of the women in my matrilineal line had what's called 'the sight.' This isn't something that only women in Traveller communities have: I believe we ALL have access to it, it's just that in my fam, it was cultivated. Now, because I have 'the sight' does it mean I'm somehow immune to fuck-ups because I can see what's unfolding? NO. But what 'the sight' *does* offer, when I get out of my own way (and THAT'S a daily bloody practice), is a deep and clear inner sight, wisdom, clarity, and discernment.

It involves being present to, recognizing, and feeling what the heart feels in real time. Which, if it's anything like mine, is total mother-loving heartbreak. AND knowing, deep in my belly and bones, that we're infinite, mother-loving, creative life force. And it's from there that I'm able to assess, discern, and respond accordingly.

And let's be clear, that's NOT easy in a world that wants us emotionally (and physically) inflamed and reactive (it's much easier to divide us and create separation that way.) You can 'see' what's going on, you can read between the words that are spoken, and hear what's not being said. You know when you're being lied to AND you know when you meet the realness in someone. For me, this is at its strongest (and most useful) during my premenstrual phase – what I call the 'Charmed and Dangerous phase.' (If you bleed, it might be worth noticing your ability to see and vision in each phase of the menstrual cycle – they WILL hold different qualities.)

Now, I rarely speak about ALL of what I see because our 'sight' does NEED discernment. Which is not to be confused with filters and taming and hiding. Discernment is our superpower because while yes, I very much want us to remember our magic, I also want us to realize and recognize that not everyone deserves it and/or is ready for it.

I repeat: This is NOT taming or hiding it. No, it's being centered, in your body and being, and using your inner sight and instincts and wisdom to witness, feel, and then respond accordingly in ANY situation AND 'see' what needs and wants to be created through you.

INVITATION:
CONNECT TO YOUR INNER VISION

Find a place where you won't be disturbed for at least half an hour. Get comfy, spray your favorite scent, and light a candle. Be sure to take in your surroundings – what's above, below, and all around you – and when you're ready, close your eyes.

1. *Call in SHE, your angels, guides, ancestors – whoever you feel most comfortable with to support and hold space for you as you activate your all-seeing 'sight.' Place your right hand on your heart and your left hand on your womb space/lower belly and take in three big, beautiful, deep breaths. In and down to your inner cauldron, your medicine bowl.*

2. *As your breath returns to its usual place and space, let yourself sink into the heaviness of your pelvic bowl. Let yourself feel strong and rooted here. When you're ready, with your left thumb, rub the spot between and above where your eyebrows meet three times in a downward direction. (Some call this spot the third eye, but ultimately, it aligns with the pineal gland in the brain.)*

3. *I then close my eyes and roll them up and in and toward that point I've just rubbed to bring my focus and attention there. I keep my breath nice and steady, and I declare my inner vision, which is actually my all-seeing vision – activated. (You don't have to do either of these practices to connect to your inner vision, but I find that if this isn't something you do daily, they're good little things to connect and ritualize the activation of your 'sight.')*

4. *Let your breath be steady, and command:* **I let myself see what needs to be seen.**

   The idea is to bring your attention to what wants to be seen in relation to a situation that you're currently experiencing. Many see this like a movie playing out. Right now, you're simply a viewer, so let yourself see what you need to see. (We're looking to build a trust in this process.) Who's present? What are they wearing?

   Now ask: What am I doing in response to this situation? And again command: I let myself see what needs to be seen.

5. *Keep this simple at first – as with anything, it's a muscle that needs to be flexed, daily if possible. When you've completed the session, with your left thumb rub the spot between and above where your eyebrows meet in a downward direction three times. Open your eyes, drink some water, and make a note of anything that wants to be remembered.*

Trust what you see

Over time, this inner vision practice can support you to become all-seeing. You'll see past and through all the ways that we've been hypnotized by fear – both personal and collective. You'll see how it's been depriving and depleting us all (on purpose) to keep us compliant. And more importantly, you'll then start to 'see' all the ways in which you can break the spell. That's when you can actively vision for YOUR/OUR future.

NOTE: If you're called, you can also pull cards – oracle, tarot, playing cards, runes; I create oracle cards with channeled art because that's an essential part of MY Wild Rose path, MY Venus story. I create them with love and color to support us all as we remember OUR magic, because divination is a powerful way to build trust with what we see.

I encourage you to find an oracle deck you love or another divination tool of your choice, and to pull daily. Keep a journal in which you riff on the message that you receive and what it means to you, and then, at the end of the day, see how that medicine/magic/message has played out FOR YOU.

BUT... you also don't NEED a divination tool. YOU are the divination tool. So, if you don't have tarot or oracle cards, or you're simply not into them, open your journal, put a hand on your heart, and ask for a word or phrase for the day. This will start to flex your knowing muscle. You let your wisdom come front and center and you then start to trust what's moving through you, what it is that you see.

You're a Source-ress, a channel, a Creatrix, and a healer. You're able to receive a dream, a possibility, a vision, and turn it into something that can heal you AND heal the Collective.

Active visioning

As I mentioned earlier, don't be surprised when the more you connect to the frequency of Venus, and the more you begin to trust what YOU see, you find that you're much less inclined to scroll through social media without intention. The Venus frequency *will* have you getting very specific about what you/we consume *visually* - in all the ways. But most importantly, you will *want* to claim autonomy over what you SEE.

Let me tell you why. (I've checked all the following deets with my husband, the Viking, because he's a nurse AND a practitioner of Ayurvedic/neuroscience/somatic health. AND he's a geek, so everything he shares is backed up and thoughtful.)

The optic nerve at the back of our eyes connects to the brain and it carries everything that we see. It runs through our pineal gland, which perceives around 12 percent of what we see and filters out what it thinks we don't need, based on what it's seen previously (it's way more complex than this, obvz). So, if you continually feed it with negativity, or bad news, or a social media scroll of 'stuff' that creates anxiety, it'll learn 'Ohh, this is normal and this is where we operate from.'

The more we feed our eyes with things that make us stress-y and anxious, the more of the stress hormone cortisol we produce. This leads to brain fog and a lack of concentration and it can pollute and disrupt our thoughts and our experience of life. However, when we choose to feed our eyes with art, beauty, things that stimulate and provoke positivity, dopamine, the happy hormone, is produced and works to help our thoughts stay clear and life feel better.

No matter what we've been led to believe, we're not simply passive participants here on Earth; we have the capacity to actively vision our ENTIRE experience. And when we vision our reality in the frequency of Venus, life becomes a LOT more delicious. And magical. It has meaning, intention, and direction. In the same way that you get to command what you see as a viewer in your mind's eye, so you're also able to visualize and reshape reality.

Again, like the affirmations, visioning – whether it's creating a vision board or doing a daily visualization practice – is often considered 'basic witch shit.' And yes, it is basic, but that's because it's foundational, AND I KNOW it works. In fact, this is HOW we create What Comes Next.

INVITATION:
ACTIVELY VISION YOUR REALITY

I don't have a five-point plan for actively visioning because it's not a one and done process. For me, it's about the daily conjuring up of my vision – Source-ress style – as if it already exists (because essentially, it does) and then actively stepping into that vision as my reality. Let's use my intention to write this book as an example:

- ❖ *I set my 'story dial' to 'void.' I actively command my subconscious to turn the dial of my stories, beliefs, and thoughts about myself as a writer/creator to 'void.' I then take a lot of deep breaths and imagine myself in the cosmic womb of NO thing and ALL possibility. A place where I am NOT who I've been told I am.*

- ❖ *I vision the scene as if it's already real. I'm a successful author who wears a red lip and expensive rose oil on her pulse points as I write. I've written a gorgeous and supportive book in the frequency of Venus. It's been received and bought with love by millions. Women carry it in their handbags (purses). They don't leave the house without it because it reminds them of their magic. They buy if for their girlfriends and host their own Wild Rose salons every Saturday afternoon to remember their magic, together.*

- ❖ *I actively CHOOSE the scene as my reality. Now, this can be a bit tricky at first, so I like to associate it with a theme tune and smell so I can use them to support me to invoke and conjure that vision (and convince my* subconscious that it is *reality*). The song is 'A Woman' by Qveen Herby and the smell is rose oil. I play the song and apply the rose oil.

❧ **I open my portable Venus altar.** *I use this as a 'spiritual' vision board, so I have a visual cue, and I then spend 10 minutes visualizing this reality. Every day.*

❧ **I affirm and activate.** *I say and write an affirmation:* **I write with ease. It's so easy for me to be creative and share my magic.**

NOTE: The act of visioning is ultimately YOU making a choice as to who you are and what you're experiencing. Don't worry about whether you're doing it right because there is no 'right' way. The idea is to make the choice to spend time in your future state and to keep meeting yourself there so that your body remembers it as known territory.

CREATE

We create our own reality by choosing to fully occupy our dreams and visions, and we do that with the moves we make and the actions we take in alignment with what we believe and perceive.

In the past, I've definitely had a tendency to dance in the dark, and let's be clear, there *is* a LOT of beauty there. AND... I've not been so good – in fact, I've been really bloody bad – at dancing in the light and have been known to be really judge-y of those who do. I'm not alone in this – there are many psychological studies that show how the percentage of time we spend in negative thought has increased and amplified, especially in the last few years. Which is why we have to CHOOSE.

We're living in times where attention is THE commodity, especially online, right? And people are doing the maddest things to get attention, saying the wildest stuff to provoke AND evoke. AND we've never been so censored. AND we've never been so narrow in our thinking, because we've been asked to put all our attention and focus on various boxes of technology and forget the magic that sits in the periphery when we broaden our vision.

So, I return to the very thing that scares them the most: US, INTENTIONALLY CHOOSING TO CREATE OUR OWN REALITY.

CHOOSING our agency and autonomy over groupthink.

CHOOSING to turn our focus toward beauty, art, and the things that light us all the way up.

CHOOSING to see, witness, explore, and experience ALL the goodness that comes when we enter life as a sensual love affair, as a feminine art form.

Vivienne Westwood kicked my arse

My heart always hurts a little more when the artists, the rebels, the creatives, the truth seekers and truth tellers (and the ones who aren't afraid to ruffle a few feathers/rock boats/challenge norms) leave Earth, but the death of fashion designer, artist, provocateur, rebel with a cause and Wild Rose Vivienne Westwood in late 2022 was to become one of the many cosmic winks/arse kicks I needed in order to choose MY Venus story.

Her very existence in the world had brought light to mine as a teen girl, and now that her light had been extinguished, it reignited a spark in me that had me turn down the dial on others' expectations of who I should be and what I should say and do all the way to zero. It was my cue to no longer simply accept what I was told is 'art' and 'truth' and instead dare to get messy, to defy the groupthink and to start making art and creating on MY terms.

In MY Venus story I make and create messy, glorious art and words from dreams and visions that have moved through me. I'm endlessly fascinated by my curiosity, and I live and love life FULL of it – source power, magic, possibility, pleasure, viriditas – so that I can be in service to love without depletion. So that I give, with all my big, beat-y heart, magic and medicine that might/might not be useful, joyful, pleasurable, and supportive to the world.

How about YOU? Consider this YOUR cosmic wink/arse kick to choose.

What reality are YOU choosing to create?

We might not be in a temple together, but we DO hold the threads/cell-deep memory of the lineage and legacy of the Wild Roses – Hathor, Isis, Mary Magdalene, Madonna, Frida Kahlo, Joan of Arc, Miley Cyrus. Invoke it now. It's Venusian. It smells like rose, myrrh, and frankincense and tastes like chocolate, honey, figs, and pomegranate seeds.

And it's waiting for you to CHOOSE. To choose yourself and to nourish, dream, visualize, and create your reality in the frequency of Venus. To choose to romance yourself and your experience of life – every last deliciously messy, juicy, dark, AND light orgasmic drop of it. Even those moments when you get triggered, feel restriction and resistance – because you will, it's how we grow. In fact, especially THOSE moments.

To choose to declare:

I am actively dreaming, visualizing, and creating MY reality. MY Venus story. So that I can experience ALL of life – the beauty AND the terror, the joy AND the pain. All the juice of life in any way I bloody desire!'

AND SO IT MOTHER LOVING IS.

 ## Follow your Wild Rose petaled path

Create your own reality
No matter what you've been led to believe, you are NOT a passive participant in life. Your reality, YOUR Venus story, is the one dreamed, created, painted, and narrated by you. Write it in as much juicy detail as you can, as if it's already true.

Make it devotional
What moves will you make and what actions will you take to stay intentional and aligned with YOUR Venus story?

All you have to do is choose
What will YOU choose?

YOU ARE A LIVING MAP OF VENUS

Choose.

Choose yourself.

Choose your body and its innate wisdom and oracular knowing.

Choose to reveal.

Your bigness.

Your magnetic and divine power.

Choose to let the beauty and wonder and romance and terror
and pain and grief and glorious magic of life consume you.

Choose to include it ALL.

This is the way of Venus.

To choose to be in your body, in your truth, in your power,
in your heart, AND in relationship with… EVERYTHING.

Live, fully alive, as a map of Venus,
revealed in plain sight.

The Empress Era: A Revolution of the Heart

*'We are entitled to wear cowboy
boots to our own revolution.'*
NAOMI WOLF

Yes, we bloody are, and a red lip too if we want. Because THIS revolution? It's OURS. It belongs to the artist, the Creatrix, the dreamer, the siren, the Source-ress – the Wild Roses. All of us who are nourished, full, and dripping with love, beauty, pleasure, and magic. All of us who are dreaming, creating, painting, and narrating realities in the frequency of Venus to restore, re-tell, and re-spell What Comes Next.

Loves, THIS is what we're here for.

To remember, reconnect with, reclaim, and revere ALL the things that have been called frivolous, distracting, and sinister. ALL the magic and medicine of Venus and her mysteries. So that we dance, sing, ritualize, nourish, and Self Source ourselves, and each other, back to life.

Back to magic.

Back to power.

Back to love.

Back to Venus.

Like the Empress in the tarot (who is a composition of ALL four queens, all four realms – material, mental, spiritual, and ethereal) we come back to our remembered magic and medicine when we align, and most importantly, harmonize, in TRUE Venusian style, all that is material, mental, spiritual, and ethereal with our big, beat-y, courageous hearts. This unlocks the Venus codes in each of us Wild Roses and fully activates the Empress in each and every one of us.

Re-telling and re-spelling the story

The Empress is soft and receptive AND fierce and feisty (and of course, like us, she's thoroughly fabulous.)

She's Venus.

She's Ma.

She's Creatrix.

She can save herself AND she knows when to ask for help.

She's a mumma, but not necessarily a mumma of children. A container – not to be tamed or kept locked away but to potentize and create healthy boundaries. A leader and a visionary, but not in an old paradigm way. She's powerful, potent, and beauty-full, but not necessarily in the conventional/beauty industry ideal. An enchantress speaking and singing and sounding the siren call of her heart with powerful intention – not for optics or attention but because it's really bloody necessary.

AND… it's the archetypal consciousness of the Empress that provides us with a mirror of ourselves, of others, of relationships, as aspects of Venus that we respect, honor, and revere as the feminine frequency. So that we're able to respect, honor, and revere them in ourselves, as ourselves.

For so long, the 'story' of Venus has been told *to* us (often by dudes) and has been shaped and formed by the culture of *Those Times*.

In *These Times* when we invoke Venus, we get to remember her as ancient-future feminine magic. We become deeply and intimately related to our bodies and our felt experience and we speak, relate, narrate, and create in the frequency of Venus. You/I/we re-spell the story and we create a revolution AND evolution with love.

Personally, I feel that our most potent power and magic is remembered in the places and spaces where we refuse to distract ourselves any longer with stories and versions and projections of who we've been told/think that we are and instead, we get deeply intimate with the FULL experience of living.

Experiencing ALL OF LIFE. The light-filled and delicious and wonder-full AND the bloody terrifying AND grief filled. We're being asked to show up for it ALL. AND… remember our magic and power (which is WAY easier to do when we're nourished and satiated and able to 'see' through the smoke and mirrors); grow strong roots (so that These Times don't shake us); and dream, visualize, and create NEW POSSIBILITIES.

Working WITH Venus is an opportunity to evaluate YOUR life, to recognize spaces and places of dissatisfaction in terms of love, relationships, beauty, worth, and values, so that you can look to create more harmony in these spaces and places THROUGH self-love and devotion. Because, and I cannot stress this enough: **More harmony in YOUR life CAN and WILL create more harmony in the world.**

It's a cell-deep devotion to the source of power within us. To the Ma of ALL creation. Our creative power is our ability to direct our attention, energy, and frequency of love. THROUGH these harmonics, we can re-tell and re-spell ALL that we've been told and sold.

Your Empress heart

The final Wild Rose I want to share with you, in this book at least, is Frances Marion, who was introduced to me by screenwriter Lauren Voloski. Frances is the woman who, according to *Time* magazine 'gave Hollywood it's voice.' Her legacy is in EVERY movie we've ever watched, yet very few people know that she was one of the US film industry's most influential screenwriters between 1915 and the late 1930s. Yep, one of the most prolific storytellers of the 20th century was a woman who, FYI, supported other women, made sure she/they got paid a shit ton of money, AND maintained creative control. WE LOVE HER.

Of course, there were continual calls to 'censor' her work, to denigrate her, and to push her out. And as we re-tell and re-spell OUR Venus story, there's a chance that they might call us/you/me delusional, insane, dangerous, crazy, and mad. It's what they've ALWAYS called anything and everything connected to women, or anyone who dares to choose love over fear, creativity over production, feels over facts, humanity over technology.

Yet – and this is Wild Rose lore, OK? – NOBODY gets to tell YOUR story except YOU. (Especially not a dude because dudes have been controlling the narrative for far too long and let's be clear, it needs a MAJOR rewrite. And especially not *anyone* who isn't living a bigger heart-led life experience than you. And FYI, I can GUARANTEE that anyone who IS living a big, heart-led life experience will be cheerleading you, NOT trying to control you.)

Look, our Wild Rose paths WILL be different. Some of us are already fully living our Venusian visions, while others are somewhere in the middle; some are excited to begin, while others may be pissed that they're not there yet. I get it. I know it might feel scary, but what's the alternative?

As I wrote this book in various locales throughout France – on MY rose line, my astrological Venus line – the French rhythm of beauty, love, and freedom became a poetic accompanying drumbeat. And as I remembered more of my magic and power, as I became the active Creatrix of MY Venus story, a strength in my physical body returned because I was clear and boundaried.

When you dance at the edges of death, you get *really* intentional about how to LIVE.

Now, I see new realities, pursue my passions, and follow my desires – unapologetically. The more I trust my response to the question 'Does this source and satiate me?' the juicier any 'yes' I choose becomes. A soft and gooey sweetness in my cynicism has appeared and it's made way for MORE magic, miracles, romance, and beauty.

Loves, WHEREVER you are on the Wild Rose path, we CAN re-tell and re-spell the story, because what I do know for SURE is that to access and be IN our magic and power, our SHE Power – Divine Feminine wisdom, the Venus frequency – we need to, on the daily, remember and reclaim who the fuck we are. Which, first and foremost, is Empress. Creatrix. Ma of ALL creation. And it's through the divine and feminine act of creation in ALL its forms in devotion to love that we call into being What Comes Next.

As Teresa of Ávila, the 16th-century nun, mystic, and *definitely* a Wild Rose said: 'The important thing is not to think much but to love much, and so do that which best awakens you to love.'

Loves, what best awakens YOU to love?

DO MORE OF IT.

Create the revolution (and evolution) direct from YOUR heart. Not by thinking, judging, or finger-pointing but by loving, much. And in these unrelentingly wild AND most magical of shifting times, I MEAN it when I say that we NEED you and your courageous, bold, and wild Empress heart (the one which, like Joan of Arc's, DID NOT/WILL NOT BURN) more than EVER.

From my Wild Rose heart to yours,

THE BIGGEST LOVE.

Closing Ceremony

As our time together closes, let the ceremony be one of the deepest devotion and reverence. A defiance of logic and information where you dare to let yourself be called 'delusional' for dreaming something entirely different to what's currently being offered as 'reality.'

Let the Egyptian mumma goddess Hathor be your guide-ess as you discover and reveal, align, define, and refine your magic, power, and true nature.

Hathor is our all-the-way-back medicine keeper of the Wild Rose path. She KNEW and still KNOWS the power of the frequency of Venus. She IS the mother-loving frequency of Venus. It's why her temples were filled with enchantresses, dreamers, music makers, and storytellers weaving and singing spells and stories to create and birth worlds and entire universes in service to love.

Call in Hathor to support you as you dream, visualize, and create YOUR Venus story. A story that WILL start revolutions of the heart throughout humanity. (You can call upon her in many ways. I've found her to love all things luxe-y – SO Venusian – but my preferred method is sipping blue-lotus and rose tea, spritzing my space with wild rose water, and shaking my sistrum.) As you build a relationship with Hathor, you'll start to discover what she digs, but to begin with, let breath and a clear intention be enough.

Breathe deep.

Deep into your belly.

Deep into your bones.

Close your eyes.

Come in.

Come down.

Into your heart.

Into your belly.

Into your pelvic bowl. Your cauldron of creation.

Let your breath return to its usual place and space as you arrive here.

Let yourself be anchored, sourced, and rooted in your center.

Let yourself, in this cauldron of creation, remember.

Remember what matters.

Hear the Wild Roses from past, present, and future chanting:

You are powerful. You are magical. You are strong. You are capable. You are love. You are full of beauty, brilliance, and the entirety of life's wonder. You are harmonious and happy. You are a Creatrix – magnetically attracting all that's in true alignment with your passion and purpose. You are BVE – Big Venus Energy.

Breathe in and let the words of the Wild Roses land in your body and being. Imagine a wild rose tightly furled at your center, and count slowly as each of the five petals, one after the other, unravels to reveal a beauty-full five-petalled wild rose in the center of your cauldron of creation. Breathe it in. It's in the frequency of Venus – it's love.

Let this frequency move through your entire body as you invite Hathor to be present in your Venus Vessel – a temple of love. She may reveal herself as a sound, a color, a sensation, or a feeling AND it may take a few times of creating this space and place before you invoke her and connect.

Breathe with her. Into your heart, into your cauldron of creation. Let her support you to remember that you DO have the capacity, through what it is that you remember, to create your destiny, to evoke, create, and fully live YOUR Venus Story.

What does that look and feel like to you?

Ask who you are, at the center of YOUR center:

What is it that I remember – that I KNOW in my body and bones wants to support me in evoking, creating, and living my Venus story?

It doesn't have to make sense – in fact, it rarely will – but let this be the question that you riff and return to often WITH Hathor.

Other Wild Roses may appear as guide-esses too. And remember that at any given moment there are Wild Roses in real time remembering that this is OUR revolution too. So, let's support each other in remembering, dreaming, visualizing, painting, creating and narrating OUR destiny. Not a meme-able, self-help-y version of 'destiny.' No, I mean our Goddess-given, Mother-loving rights and rites – of power, of magic, and of creating (entire bloody universes if we want to) in service to love. OUR VENUS STORY.

AND SO IT MOTHER-LOVING IS.

Acknowledgments

France – for being the very best teacher of *my* Venusian mysteries.

The SHE Power Collective – for supporting me and trusting me. I love that we're all in process (and progress) together.

The hot Viking, Rich – for your big heart, your love of *this* Wild Rose, and for always being ready and available for EVERY adventure. I LOVE you and I LOVE the Venus story that *we* create, shape, paint, and narrate together.

Sarah – for being the most incredible techno witch, supporter, gift buyer, and friend. Thanks for always being on my team.

Kay and Ron – you beauty-full, big-hearted humans. Thanks for always giving us a home in France, for sharing your animals, and for being the most gorgeous friends. We're blessed.

Leanne, Sarah, Nicholas, Katie, and David – cheerleaders, food sharers, word wranglers, tear wipers, laughter makers, each with the ability to have two-hour-minimum phone convos. I bloody LOVE YOU.

Simon, Psio, and Mo – the three wise men. Thank you for your medicine, laughter, wisdom, and care. You don't know each other, but you're three very powerful and trusted medicine men supporting *this* Wild Rose and for that I'm VERY grateful. Honoring and celebrating you!

The Hay House team – THANK YOU to everyone involved in turning *Venus* from an idea into a hold-in-your-hand book. With special thanks to Michelle Pilley for believing in and commissioning MY Venus story, and the Editrix queens, Amy, Debra, and Grace: You are *quite* the trifecta!

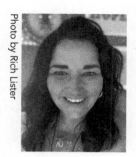

About the Author

Lisa Lister is a best-selling author, artist, well-woman therapist, somatic movement teacher and practitioner, and a Movement in Practice facilitator.

She offers support, space, remembrance, spiritual guidance, astrological insight, cyclical maps, and counsel to women who are exploring, navigating, and wanting to heal their relationship with their body, power, sex, creativity, pleasure, and passion in these 'interesting' times.

She has a BIG love for: maximalism – all the color, all the things. Everything French – EVERYTHING. A red lip – her main life quest is for the perfect shade: not too orange, with a hint of blue, heading more toward raspberry; if you know of one, hook her up with it. Stationery – inky pens and Louise Carmen Paris notebooks; beauty-full. Romance novels – she has proof that love and happy-ever-afters do exist, because she's creating and living it.

www.thesassyshe.com